11-30-59

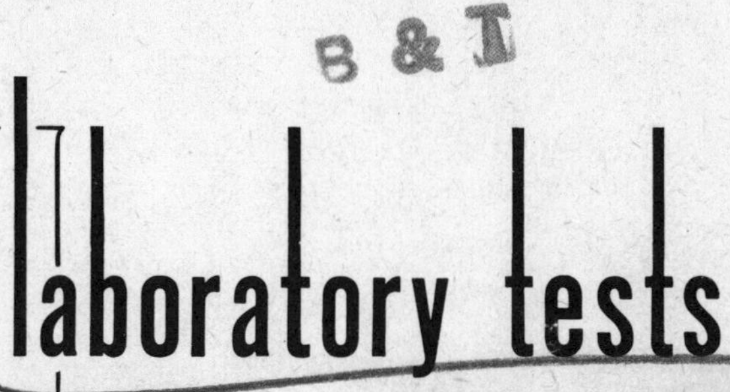

laboratory tests
IN COMMON USE

by **SOLOMON GARB, M.D.**

Associate Professor of Pharmacology,
Albany Medical College

SECOND EDITION

SPRINGER Publishing Company, Inc.
New York, N.Y.

SPRINGER PUBLISHING COMPANY, INC.
44 East 23rd Street New York 10, N.Y.

Second Edition
First printing, September 1959

First Edition

First printing, April 1956
Second printing, August 1956
Third printing, January 1957
Fourth printing, April 1957
Fifth printing, March 1958
Sixth printing, January 1959

Price: $2.50 (*Send payment with order for single copy*)
Quantity price: 10 or more copies, $2.25 each

Library of Congress Catalog Card Number: 59-14847

Printed in U.S.A.

Preface to the Second Edition

This edition has been brought up to date by the addition of ten laboratory tests, several tables, and other material. In deciding which of the newer tests to include, I have been aided greatly by nurses throughout the country, who wrote suggesting changes and additions which would increase the usefulness of the book. Reviews of the first edition were also read carefully, and changes were made to conform to justifiable criticism; for example, the chapter "Normal Values in Infants and Children" was added.

The new edition continues the practice of emphasizing those aspects of the tests with which the nurse is most concerned, while summarizing briefly the technical laboratory procedures.

September 1959 S. G.

Preface to the First Edition

The idea for this book grew out of a course that I taught at Hunter College on problems in physiology for nurses. Much of the course dealt with the physiological significance of laboratory tests. The students—graduate nurses working toward a degree in nursing education—felt that an understanding of the reasons for ordering such tests and an idea of how the tests aid in the diagnosis and management of the patient is important in nursing; they also pointed out the need for a brief book on the meaning of laboratory tests.

The book has therefore been written primarily for the nurse, the graduate as well as the student. It is hoped that it will also prove useful to the laboratory technician, medical secretary, and medical student, and become a convenient source of practical information for the physician.

In class room teaching, it is helpful to group laboratory tests according to the specimens employed (blood, urine, etc.) *and* according to the organ or system whose function is to be measured. I felt that the book, too, should offer the two points of view. The descriptive part of the book is arranged according to the *specimens employed* in tests. A series of tables provides the complementary information according to *organs whose function is tested.*

The aspects with which the nurse is most directly concerned are fully described for each test, while other information is summarized. The purpose of each test is given in sufficient detail to enable the reader to understand why the test was ordered and what the results may signify. The procedure for collecting the specimen is described in such a manner that the nurse can collect and send to the laboratory the correct specimen; laboratory procedures are briefly stated in general terms. The procedures included are those I believe to be most commonly in use. However, no inference should be drawn that these are necessarily preferred in a particular hospital or institution.

I am grateful to my students and colleagues whose comments and suggestions helped shape this volume; to Dr. Walter Modell who gave me many valuable suggestions based on his experience as writer and teacher; and to Miss Ida Dailes for her efficient secretarial and editorial help.

Contents

1

Introduction

Laboratory tests aid in the diagnosis and management of various disorders. Only those in relatively common use are included in this book. A test may be ordered by a physician to confirm his suspicion or impression, or it may be performed routinely on most or all patients. Routine tests are carried out because the disorders they demonstrate are relatively common and the tests themselves relatively easy and inexpensive to perform. An example of this sort of test is the determination of blood hemoglobin concentration. A substantial proportion of the population has anemia, so that this test, performed on 100 patients with complaints not related to the blood, will reveal several who would benefit from anti-anemia therapy. Hemoglobin, serology and urinalysis examinations are performed routinely on most patients. Many physicians and hospitals also include a complete blood count, guaiac test of the feces, chest x-ray, and an electrocardiogram.

Some tests have no significance other than to indicate the diagnosis. An example of this is the glucose tolerance test. Should the result of such a test indicate the presence of diabetes, the test is of no further use in regulating treatment. Many tests, however, can be useful in following the course of the disease or in adjusting therapy. An example of the latter is the test for prothrombin time. In treatment with Dicumarol and similar drugs, tests for prothrombin time are performed daily to aid in prescribing the correct dose of Dicumarol for the current day.

In some institutions a single laboratory performs all the tests; in others there may be several laboratories, one performing bacteriological tests, another chemical tests, and so on.

The origin of the test material does not always correspond to the organ or system being examined. A test may be performed on urine to obtain information on liver function. Since, in the following chapters, the tests are arranged according to the type of specimen examined (i.e., blood, urine, etc.), a supplementary listing is included (Chapter 9) which groups the tests according to the organ or system whose functions are being tested.

It should be noted that many of the tests are useful in diagnosing diseases of more than one organ or system. This, of course, is a natural consequence of the interrelationship between the various organs and systems of the body. In many cases, therefore, the interpretation of the results of these tests by the physician is not simply a matter of routine but involves careful integration with history and physical findings.

In some cases the relationship of a laboratory test to the pathological physiology of a disease is clear. For example, since the kidney excretes urea, it might be predicted that in advanced kidney disease the blood urea levels will be elevated. On the other hand, the exact relationship of some laboratory tests to the pathological physiology of disease is not known. An example of this is the thymol turbidity test for liver function. In these cases it has been found empirically that the tests are usually positive in certain types of disorders. There are theories which attempt to correlate the test results with the disease process, but since they are unproven, and in most cases highly complex, they are not discussed in this book.

There are other tests, such as the determination of the sedimentation rate, which are so non-specific that they do not point to any particular group of diseases, but only indicate that there is some disorder.

As additional aids Chapters 8, 10, 11 and 12 are included.

Chapter 8 summarizes the important distinctions to be made between normal values for adults, and for infants and children.

The first six tables of Chapter 10 are designed for quick reference for the nurse on duty who needs to know how much blood or other material is required for a particular test, whether anticoagulant is added, and what type of container is to be used. Normal ranges for adults are included in these tables. Table 7 lists drugs and diagnostic agents which contain iodine, and which would confuse the interpretation of several thyroid-function tests. Table 8 lists most of the currently available laboratory aids and materials for rapid, simplified laboratory tests. Through the judicious use of these materials, diagnostic tests may often be performed more rapidly, conveniently and economically.

Chapter 11 consists of a description of the units of measurement used in clinical laboratory procedures.

Chapter 12 summarizes the principal rules that apply to the care of needles and syringes and to the technique of venipuncture.

PART ONE: TESTS

according to type of specimen employed

2

Bacteriological Tests

Materials collected for bacteriological examination fall into two groups: (1) Cultures made at the bedside, and (2) Specimens to be cultured in the laboratory.

A *culture* consists of material inoculated directly into a culture medium. In most hospitals only nose and throat secretions and venous blood are put into culture media at the bedside. The culture should be placed in an incubator at once, so that the bacteria may grow.

A *specimen* consists of material which will be cultured in the laboratory. All bacteriological specimens, other than spinal fluid, are kept in the bacteriological refrigerator to preserve the organisms. Spinal fluid may contain organisms which are sensitive to cold and is therefore placed in a bacteriological incubator.

In handling specimens and cultures for bacteriological examinations, it is at all times essential to keep in mind the possible danger of spreading infectious agents. All persons handling bacteriological material must know the necessary protective procedures. It is also important that the specimens reach the laboratory in a condition suitable for culture. Accordingly, the following precautions must be observed:

1. Use standard equipment. Do not substitute other containers for those designated by the laboratory.
2. Do not use cracked or broken containers.
3. Use only the regulation plugs to stopper tubes and bottles. Do not substitute gauze, paper, ordinary cotton, or other materials.
4. Do not use applicators which are broken or in any way contaminated.
5. Use only one applicator per tube.
6. Do not use Petri dishes for specimens which are fluid or which ooze fluids, including blood, except in bedside blood cultures.
7. Remove plugs from containers gently, with a twisting motion; do not pull straight out.
8. Discard any plug which comes in contact with an unsterile surface.
9. Do not fill containers more than half-way.
10. Do not allow plugs to become wet, either from the specimen or from other sources. Wet plugs may contaminate personnel handling them and may also contaminate the specimen.
11. Do not spill any material on the outside of containers, plugs, boxes, tables, etc. If such material is spilled accidentally, call the bacteriology laboratory to find out how best to destroy the infectious agent. Ordinary soap and water may not be adequate. Do not allow anyone to come near the spilled material.
12. Make sure that plugs are firmly in place when the procedure is completed.
13. Plugs should be rotated clockwise.

14. Specimens and cultures should be carried in an upright position, and should not be shaken.
15. After collection, the specimen should be sent to the laboratory at once.
16. Certain organisms such as the gonococcus, and the Pertussis and Brucella groups need freshly prepared culture media. Therefore, if the presence of these organisms is suspected, the laboratory must be notified at least an hour before the specimen is collected.

Agglutination Tests

The blood is tested for substances made by the body to neutralize a particular invading organism. These substances, known as agglutinins, cause such microorganisms to clump together. When specific agglutinins are present, they indicate that the body has been exposed to the microorganism in question and has developed some immunity to it. This procedure can be used with a large variety of microorganisms. However, only three groups are usually tested for in most laboratories in this country. They are:

1. The Brucella, or undulant fever, group of bacteria.
2. The typhoid and paratyphoid group of bacteria. This is called the Widal test.
3. Rickettsia. This agglutination reaction differs from the others in that the organism which is agglutinated is not the rickettsia itself but a bacterium, Proteus OX19, which for some unknown reason is agglutinated by the anti-rickettsial agglutinins. This test is also known as the Weil-Felix test.

There is an important consideration in judging the results of these tests. A positive test indicates only that the patient harbored the microorganism *at some time;* it does not necessarily indicate that the organism is still present. A patient who had the suspected disease years previously may still have a positive agglutination reaction.

Procedure for Collecting Specimen. Venous blood is withdrawn, 5 cc. placed in a test tube and allowed to coagulate. The tests are performed on the serum. The quantity is sufficient for all three agglutination tests. Particular care must be exercised to prevent the spilling of blood on the outside of the test tube since blood frequently contains virulent organisms.

Laboratory Procedure. The laboratory adds serial dilutions of the patient's serum to suspensions of either live or killed bacteria. Observations are then made, sometimes with and sometimes without a microscope, to see whether clumping has occurred and to determine the range of dilutions within which the agglutination takes place. The dilutions ordinarily used range up to 1:1024. When live bacteria are used, they remain virulent when agglutinated and must be disposed of carefully.

Normal Range. Normal people sometimes have small amounts of agglutinin in their blood. Accordingly, the lowest concentration of the serum at which agglutination takes place is important. In the Widal test for typhoid fever, a positive agglutination at concentrations of 1:40 or 1:80 and up is required for a definite diagnosis.

In the diagnosis of brucellosis by agglutination, a positive response at a serum dilution of 1:50 to 1:100 or over is required, depending on the skin test.

In the Weil-Felix test for rickettsial disease, agglutination must take place at serum dilutions of 1:50 or more for the test to be positive.

If there is doubt as to whether a positive agglutination test comes from a current infection or an earlier one, repeated tests may be performed at intervals of 3 to 5 days. Agglutination in progressively weaker dilutions of serum strongly suggests a current infection.

Antibiotic Sensitivity Test

It is sometimes important to know which antibiotic is most effective against a particular strain of bacteria causing a patient's illness. This can sometimes be determined in the laboratory, using the disc or tube dilution methods. Since there are many variables which determine the effectiveness of antibiotics, these tests are only suggestive.

Procedure for Collecting Specimen. The same as for corresponding cultures.

Laboratory Procedure. The ability of various antibiotics to stop or slow the multiplication of bacteria is measured. There are several methods which may be used. The most common of these is the disc method which involves placing small discs of filter paper containing an antibiotic on a Petri dish streaked with a culture of the bacteria. The width of the zone of growth inhibition around the disc determines the sensitivity of the organism to the antibiotic. In the tube dilution method, the bacteria are cultured in a series of tubes containing known concentrations of an antibiotic. The lowest concentration completely inhibiting multiplication of the bacteria determines the sensitivity of the organism.

Blood Culture

Many varieties of bacteria may produce bacteremia or bloodstream infections. Frequently, a precise identification of the offending microorganism is necessary to enable the physician to select the appropriate antibiotic. Some types of bacteria do not survive changes in temperature or prolonged standing in the absence of special culture media, so that it is impractical to send a specimen of venous blood to be cultured. The procedure, therefore, is carried out at the bedside. Since different kinds of bacteria require different conditions in order to multiply, several types of media are used.

Precaution. Doctor, nurse, and patient must wear masks to avoid contamination of the culture.

Materials. A blood culture set usually consists of the following:

a. Two Petri dishes.
b. One bottle of infusion broth with glucose.
c. One bottle of plain infusion broth, which may have penicillinase added if the patient has received penicillin.
d. Two tubes of agar.

Procedure for Collecting Specimen. The following steps are taken:

1. The stoppered tubes of agar are heated in a container of boiling water until the material is completely liquified.
2. Place the tubes of agar in a container of water at 50° C. *as measured with a thermometer.* If the temperature falls below 45° C. the agar will solidify and have to be remelted. If the temperature is above 50° C. the bacteria may be destroyed.
3. Prepare the patient's skin at the site of venipuncture with a suitable antiseptic (benzylkonium chloride) and draw 13 cc. of blood into a sterile syringe.
4. Place 5 cc. of blood in each bottle of broth.
5. Place 1 cc. of blood in one Petri dish and 2 cc. in the other.
6. Add the agar at 50° C. to the blood and cover the Petri dishes. Rotate gently, without splashing, to mix uniformly.
7. Allow the agar in the Petri dish to solidify for *at least 10 minutes.* Then invert and place flat.
8. Label each container with name and location of patient, and *date* and *hour* when the culture was made.
9. Deliver the cultures to the laboratory or place them in the bacteriological incubator.

Laboratory Procedure. The laboratory will observe the cultures at regular intervals. If bacteriological growth appears, they will endeavor to identify the organism by direct smears. Frequently they will have to make one or more subcultures for positive identification. Final reports may therefore be delayed as long as 10 days. Usually, however, preliminary reports on blood cultures are available after 36 hours.

Normal Range. Normal blood should be sterile. Any microorganism found in the blood culture is either a contaminant from an imperfect procedure or indicates a pathological condition.

Dark-Field Examination

This is a variety of bacteriological examination which is usually done to determine whether the Treponema of syphilis is present. The test is performed on fluid oozing out of lesions of skin or mucous membranes, not on blood. This special type of examination is needed because the Treponema is too thin to be seen by ordinary microscopic techniques, but can be seen by reflected light in a dark field.

Procedure for Collecting Specimen. The specimen is collected by the person (usually a bacteriologist or pathologist) doing the examination. In most institutions the patient is brought to the laboratory for this examination.

Precaution. Material from a dark-field positive lesion is highly infectious. All personnel who may come in contact with it should be protected.

Laboratory Procedure. The material is examined in a dark field for the Treponema pallidum. Careful observation is needed to distinguish the Treponema pallidum from similar forms which are normally found in the mouth, and which do not cause disease.

Normal Range. Normally there are no Treponema pallidum to be seen.

Miscellaneous Fluid Cultures

Various body cavities sometimes fill with fluid which may contain bacteria. The pleural, peritoneal and pericardial cavities are most commonly involved.

Procedure for Collecting Specimen. The physician removes the specimen and places it in a sterile tube, using aseptic technique.

Laboratory Procedure. Essentially the same as in blood culture test.

Normal Range. Normally these body cavities are sterile. Therefore, any bacteria found in the culture are either pathogenic or contaminants resulting from an imperfect collection procedure.

Nose and Throat Culture

It is frequently useful for the physician to know which bacteria are present in the nose and throat. This information is obtained by means of a nose and throat culture.

Procedure for Collecting Specimen. The physician collects the specimen on a sterile cotton swab. The swab is suspended in a sterile culture tube containing 2 cc. of broth, *without touching the broth.* The broth is not a culture medium. It is used to keep the air around the swab moist so that evaporation and drying of the specimen does not occur. Special culture tubes containing Loeffler's medium are used when diphtheria is suspected. In the latter case, the medium does touch the swab.

Laboratory Procedure. The swab will be plated (streaked gently across a Petri dish containing agar) . The colonies that grow out will then be identified microscopically or, if necessary, subcultures will be made.

Normal Range. Many bacteria are normally found in the nose and throat, including pneumococci, staphylococci, streptococci, H. influenzae, K. pneumoniae, and others. The decision as to whether a particular type found in the culture is related to the patient's illness can usually be made only after the physician has correlated these and other findings. Certain types of bacteria, such as those causing tuberculosis or diphtheria, are always abnormal.

Spinal Fluid Culture

The spinal fluid is examined in cases of suspected meningitis. There are several kinds of microorganisms which may produce meningitis and precise identification is usually important in order that the most suitable antibiotic may be selected.

Procedure for Collecting Specimen. The physician places 2 cc. of spinal fluid in a special small test tube. The specimen is stored in an incubator, not a refrigerator.

Laboratory Procedure. This is the same as in other

cultures. Because of the urgency that exists in the case of meningitis, the laboratory will call the floor as soon as the organism has been identified.

Normal Range. The spinal fluid is normally sterile.

Sputum Culture

Sputum is material brought up from the lungs and trachea during deep coughing. It should not be confused with saliva or post-nasal secretions. This test is often of value in diagnosing lung infections. Since sputum is often contaminated with postnasal secretions and saliva, the organisms found in these secretions may also occur in sputum cultures.

Procedure for Collecting Specimen. The patient uses a special specimen cup or box with a cover. He is instructed to place the sputum raised by a few good coughs into the container. The container is delivered without delay to the bacteriology refrigerator. Containers holding sputum should not be allowed to remain at the bedside for hours. The patient must be warned not to get any sputum on the outside of the container, and it should never be completely filled. If the patient is on isolation, the outside of the container is contaminated and must be handled with the necessary technique to avoid spreading infection.

Laboratory Procedure. Essentially the same as with other cultures with special attention to the presence of acid-fast (tubercle) bacilli.

Normal Range. Both pathogenic and nonpathogenic bacteria are found in some lung diseases. The physician, therefore, after correlating all his findings must decide whether a particular finding is likely to be significant.

Stool Culture

The normal bacterial flora of the stool are the largest in number and kind found in any part of the body. About 50 varieties of bacteria are normally present in the stool. There are also several kinds of pathogenic bacteria. Different culture media are needed for some of the pathogenic bacteria. The laboratory, therefore, should always be told which bacteria to look for.

Procedure for Collecting Specimen. Use special containers with properly fitted covers. Use a tongue depressor to place a small amount of feces (about 1 inch in diameter) into the container. Avoid contaminating the outside of the container. Deliver promptly to the bacteriology laboratory or refrigerator. Specimens obtained at proctoscopy may be collected on swabs, as described in *Nose and Throat Culture.*

Laboratory Procedure. This will depend on the type of pathogenic bacteria suspected.

Normal Range. About 50 types of bacteria are normally present in the feces. Some not normally found may be harmless. Usually, specific pathogens such as those of typhoid, dysentery, brucellosis, etc., are sought for and reported if present.

Tests for Special Microorganisms

Certain tests for virus and rickettsial diseases are not ordinarily performed in the hospital laboratory but are sent to a public health department laboratory. In large city health departments or in state public health laboratories, tests may be performed for many diseases, including Colorado tick fever, influenza, mumps, psittacosis, Q-fever, typhus, and several kinds of virus encephalitis. Tests may also be performed for parasitic infestations such as amebiasis, trichinosis, and echinococcosis. Certain other diseases are tested for by the United States Public Health Laboratory, such as trypanosomiasis, schistosomiasis, filariasis, leishmaniasis, histoplasmosis, blastomycosis, toxoplasmosis, and leptospirosis.

Procedure for Collecting Specimen. Two specimens of blood are required. One is drawn during the acute phase of the disease and the other two weeks later. About 10 cc. of blood is placed in a test tube and allowed to coagulate. The specimen, needle and syringe are handled with great care to avoid contamination of personnel with infectious agents. Packing of the sample for shipment to the appropriate laboratory is done according to the directions of that laboratory. Special containers may usually be obtained from the hospital laboratory.

Urine Culture

Urine culture is often of value in determining the etiological agent in infectious diseases of kidneys, ureters and bladder.

Procedure for Collecting Specimen. In some cases it is possible to collect a sterile noncatheterized specimen from men after cleaning the genital area. However, even with all precautions, some contamination may occur. Therefore, noncatheterized specimens must be brought to the bacteriology laboratory at once, before the contaminating microorganisms multiply and crowd out the pathogens sought. For women patients it has been customary to use catheterized specimens only. However, recent studies have questioned this procedure. It has been shown that, despite all precautions, the insertion of a catheter into the bladder often introduces infection. *Accordingly, many doctors now believe that it is too risky to catheterize women patients for urine culture.* Instead, a clean, voided specimen is used. The entire vulvar area is carefully cleansed, using benzalkonium (Zephiran). The labia are held apart and urine is voided into a sterile bottle. The urine culture is often contaminated by skin bacteria but contamination of the culture is preferable to contamination of the bladder. It is essential to note on the chart whether the urine specimen is passed normally or via catheter.

Laboratory Procedure. Essentially the same as in other ypes of culture.

Normal Range. Normal urine is sterile. Any bacteria found are contaminants from the skin, or invading organisms.

Weil-Felix Test—*See Agglutination Tests*

Widal Test

See Agglutination Tests

Wound Culture

When wounds or surgical incisions show evidence of infection, it is frequently important to identify the invading organism so that specific therapy may be instituted.

Procedure for Collecting Specimen. The physician collects pus or exudate from the wound on a sterile cotton swab. The swab is placed in a sterile tube as described under *Nose and Throat Culture.*

Laboratory Procedure. The laboratory procedure is generally similar to other cultures. However, special efforts are made to culture anaerobic bacteria, since their presence is serious and requires special handling.

Normal Range. All wounds and surgical incisions are contaminated by bacteria. However, only a small proportion of them are actually infected. The significance of a culture, therefore, depends on the type of microorganism found and on the clinical picture. Normal skin flora include diphtheroids, E. coli, B. subtilis, P. vulgaris, streptococci, and staphylococci, but others are also found.

3

Tests Performed on Blood

Many tests are performed on blood for diagnostic purposes. When only a drop or two of blood is needed for a test, such as a hemoglobin determination or white blood cell count, it is usually obtained by pricking the finger or ear lobe. This blood oozes from capillaries and is, therefore, called capillary blood. When a larger quantity is needed, it is obtained from a vein and is called venous blood.

The accuracy of these determinations usually depends less on the laboratory procedures than on the method of collecting and transporting the specimen. Improper handling of the specimen may give erroneous and misleading results. It is thus essential that in collecting blood for the laboratory the following precautions be observed:

1. The patient must be in the fasting state unless otherwise specified. Absorption of food may alter many of the blood constituents. If fats are absorbed, their presence in the blood (lipemia) may interfere with some tests such as bilirubin, albumin-globulin ratio, and others. The patient may have water.
2. Hemolysis will cause serious errors in many tests

such as those for potassium, serum bilirubin, and others. This can be avoided by observing the following precautions:

a. The syringe must be perfectly dry as well as sterile, since ordinary water will hemolyze red cells.
b. When drawing the blood, an even pressure should be used in pulling back the plunger of the syringe. Avoid excessive negative pressure.
c. After drawing the blood, remove the needle from the syringe and empty the latter into the correct container without foaming or splashing the blood.
d. Do not use containers which have been chilled.
e. Avoid shaking the specimen unnecessarily.

3. If the patient is receiving an intravenous infusion in one arm, blood should be drawn from the other arm to avoid contamination or dilution of the specimen.
4. Concentration of the blood through venous stasis should be prevented, or some of the tests will give inaccurrate results. In order to avoid this, the tourniquet should be removed from the arm after the needle is definitely in the vein. Allow several seconds to elapse while fresh venous blood fills the vein; then draw the blood into the syringe. Unfortunately, this precaution is ignored by many physicians and nurses. As a result some of the determinations on blood samples drawn by them are inaccurate. The correct procedure is simple and

only requires an additional fraction of a minute.
5. After specimens are drawn, they should be sent to the laboratory as soon as possible. If the determinations cannot be made at once, the laboratory is responsible for handling or treating the specimen so that it may be stored safely.

Most tests are designated as "routine." That is, they are performed by the laboratory in the ordinary working schedule, since there is no important medical advantage in having the results available before late afternoon or the following day. In a few cases it may be necessary to know the results of a particular test as soon as possible. Such specimens are labeled "emergency" and the test is carried out at once. The "emergency" designation is the responsibility of the physician in charge and should be made only for genuine medical reasons. It is improper to designate a test as an emergency in order to facilitate a patient's early discharge or because the sample was drawn too late for routine testing that day.

Only the following tests are likely to be designated as emergencies: amylase, urea nitrogen (B.U.N.), CO_2 combining power, potassium, prothrombin, sodium, sugar, and determination of blood types.

When blood or other fluids, known or suspected to be harboring a microorganism causing infectious disease, are sent for other than bacteriological examination, the specimen should be labeled in red "Infectious Material." Examples are: blood, urine and stools from typhoid patients; spinal fluid in meningitis; and blood in various rickettsial and virus diseases.

At times, a large number of blood determinations are ordered for a patient on a single day. If the total amount of blood needed for all tests exceeds 20 cc. it may prove difficult, or impossible, to obtain it from a patient with poor circulation. In that case the laboratory can often manage to perform a satisfactory test with less blood than is usually requested. It is advisable to call the laboratory beforehand and ask whether this can be done with the series of tests ordered.

A/G (Albumin-Globulin) Ratio

See Albumin, Globulin, Total Protein, A/G Ratio

Acid Phosphatase

—*See Phosphatase, Acid*

Albumin, Globulin, Total Protein, and A/G Ratio

These tests are usually performed together. They may be useful in the diagnosis of kidney, liver, and some other diseases.

The main function of the serum albumin appears to be the maintenance of osmotic pressure of the blood. The main function of serum globulin is not fully understood, but one of its secondary functions is to assist in maintaining the osmotic pressure of the blood. Since the globulin molecule is several times as large as the albumin molecule it is less efficient, gram for gram, in maintaining osmotic pressure. In certain diseases the albumin may leak out of capillary walls, while the larger globulin molecules are retained within the blood stream. The body may then compensate for loss of albumin by producing more globulin, so that the globulin becomes responsible for a larger share of the osmotic pressure. Yet despite normal or even increased total dissolved protein in the serum, osmotic pressure may be less than normal because of the lesser effectiveness of globulin. As a result there may be some edema. By discovering a shift in the albumin-globulin ratio, the physician is aided in diagnosing the patient's illness. He may also rely on repeated albumin-globulin ratio determinations for judging the effectiveness of treatment.

Conditions in which the albumin-globulin ratio is lowered include chronic nephritis, lipoid nephrosis, liver disease, amyloid nephrosis, and malnutrition.

Procedure for Collecting Specimen. Venous blood is withdrawn and 6 cc. placed in a test tube and allowed to coagulate. The test is performed on the serum.

Laboratory Procedure. The total protein in a sample of serum is determined by the Kjeldahl method. Then the albumin is separated from another sample of serum and the amount measured. The concentration of globulin is determined by subtracting the value for albumin from the total protein.

Normal Range. Total serum protein, 6.0 to 8.0 Gm. per 100 cc. of serum; serum albumin, 3.2 to 5.6 Gm. per 100 cc. of serum; serum globulin, 1.3 to 3.2 Gm. per 100 cc. of serum; A/G ratio, 1.5:1 to 2.5:1.

Alkaline Phosphatase —*See Phosphatase, Alkaline*

Amylase

In certain types of pancreatic disease, the digestive encymes of the pancreas escape into the surrounding tissue, producing necrosis with severe pain and inflammation. Under these circumstances there is an increase in the serum amylase. A serum amylase level of twice normal usually indicates acute pancreatitis. However, there are times when the serum amylase is elevated in abdominal conditions, such as intestinal obstruction.

Some surgeons order routine serum amylase tests for the first few days after any operation which might have injured the pancreas. Whenever an elevation in the amylase level is found, they can institute therapy for pancreatitis early, thus increasing the patient's chances for recovery.

This test remains positive for a short time only, seldom for more than a few days.

Procedure for Collecting Specimen. Venous blood is withdrawn and a 6 cc. sample allowed to coagulate in a test tube. At times this test may be designated "emergency" by the physician.

Laboratory Procedure. The speed with which 1 cc. of serum digests a starch solution to erythrodextrins (intermediate products of starch digestion) is measured by means of an iodine color reaction.

Normal Range. 80 to 150 units (Somogyi).

Anti-Streptolysin O Titer

This test, usually used in suspected rheumatic fever, indicates the reaction of the body to a recent streptococcal infection. The streptococcus produces many enzymes, one of which, streptolysin O, has the ability to destroy red blood corpuscles. Part of the defense against this bacterium is an antibody which neutralizes streptolysin. Since rheumatic fever is related to a recent streptococcal infection, an increase in the titer of the anti-streptolysin is usually found in rheumatic fever. It should be clear, however, that this test, like all others useful in rheumatic fever, is non-specific and can be positive in many other conditions.

Infants and young children sometimes have normal anti-streptolysin titers despite clear-cut rheumatic fever.

Procedure for Collecting Specimen. Venous blood is withdrawn and 5 cc. placed in a test tube and allowed to clot. The test is performed on the serum.

Laboratory Procedure. A purified streptolysin from a streptococcus culture is standardized for its ability to dissolve rabbit red blood cells in suspension. Serial dilutions of the patient's serum are then tested to determine the greatest dilution which will prevent this effect of streptolysin.

Normal Range. Up to 200 units per cc. of serum.

Ascorbic Acid (Vitamin C)

Ascorbic acid is an essential vitamin found in fresh fruits and vegetables. Severe deficiencies in ascorbic acid cause scurvy which is usually readily recognized. However, moderate deficiencies are fairly common and may cause subclinical scurvy, not readily recognized. It is manifested by weakness, anemia, lowered resistance to infection, and delayed healing of wounds. A low blood level of ascorbic acid establishes a diagnosis of the deficiency.

Procedure for Collecting Specimen. Venous blood is withdrawn and a 6 cc. sample placed in an oxalate bottle. The test is performed on plasma pipetted from the sample.

Laboratory Procedure. Several different methods are available. Most of them are based on the ability of ascorbic acid to decolorize a solution made blue by the addition of a special reagent.

Normal Range. 0.7 to 1.4 Gm. per 100 cc. of blood plasma.

Bilirubin, Partition (Direct and Indirect van den Bergh Test)

When the ability of the liver to excrete bilirubin is impaired by obstruction, either within or outside the organ, it is believed that the excess circulating bilirubin is free of any attached protein. However, when the increase in circulating bilirubin is due to increased destruction of red blood cells (hemolysis), it is believed that the bilirubin is bound to protein. By measuring the amount of free bilirubin (direct) and the amount bound to protein (indirect), there is some indication as to whether the patient's illness is based on obstruction or hemolysis.

Procedure for Collecting Specimen. Venous blood is withdrawn and 5 cc. placed in a test tube and allowed to coagulate. The test is performed on the serum, but it is also possible to use plasma separated from uncoagulated blood.

Laboratory Procedure. The direct method is described below. In the indirect method alcohol is added to the sample of serum. The serum proteins precipitate, freeing any bilirubin which was bound to them, and the bilirubin dissolves in the alcohol. Ehrlich's reagent is then added to the alcoholic extract and the intensity of the color produced is measured.

Normal Range. 0.1 to 1.0 mg. per 100 cc. Within the normal range there is no significance to the ratio between the amounts of bilirubin found on direct and indirect measurements. When the concentration of bilirubin rises significantly over 1.0 mg. per 100 cc., the relative amounts which are free and bound to protein may suggest the type of disorder. If most of the bilirubin is found on the direct test, the chances are that the patient has an obstructive lesion. If most of it is found on the indirect test, the illness is likely to be hemolytic. These interpretations indicate probabilities, not certainties, and there is some controversy about the meaning of these tests.

Bilirubin, Total

Bilirubin is derived from the hemoglobin in red blood cells which have been broken down. It is constantly being produced, and is excreted by the liver into the bile, of which it is the chief pigment. There is always a small amount in the serum. When the destruction of red blood cells becomes excessive or when the liver is unable to excrete the ordinary quantities of bilirubin produced, the concentration in the serum rises. If the concentration becomes very high, there is visible jaundice. It is advantageous to discover the increased concentration of serum bilirubin before jaundice is seen, and that is accomplished by this test.

Procedure for Collecting Specimen. Venous blood is withdrawn and 5 cc. placed in a test tube and allowed to coagulate. The test is performed on the serum but it is also possible to use plasma separated from uncoagulated blood.

Laboratory Procedure. To the sample of serum is added Ehrlich's reagent. A colored product is formed and the intensity of the color is used as a measure of the bilirubin concentration.

Normal Range. 0.1 to 1.0 mg. per 100 cc. of serum.

Bleeding Time

This test measures the time during which there is bleeding from a small skin incision. It is quite distinct from tests for clotting time and gives somewhat different information since, in a bleeding time test, constriction of the small vessels is also involved. Bleeding time is prolonged in thrombocytopenic purpura and other blood disorders.

Procedure for Performing Test and Collecting Specimen. A standardized puncture wound of the skin is produced with an appropriate instrument. The site of the puncture may be the finger tip, ear lobe, or forearm. In some variations when the arm is used, a blood pressure cuff increases the venous pressure to make the test more sensitive. After the puncture is produced, the drops of blood are wiped away with filter paper every 30 seconds. The time at which bleeding stops is recorded.

Normal Range. 1 to 6 minutes.

Blood Counts

Frequently, various blood cell and platelet counts are ordered either routinely to help with a particular problem, or to follow the results of treatment. Several counts are often performed together and will, therefore, be considered together here. Blood counts are performed on whole blood, usually capillary blood, although venous blood can be used.

Platelet Count

The platelets (thrombocytes), which are necessary for the clotting of blood, are particles much smaller than red blood cells. They are reduced in such conditions as thrombocytopenic purpura, aplastic anemia, Goucher's disease, and septicemia. They may be increased in polycythemia, fractures, and certain kinds of anemia.

Procedure for Performing Test and Collecting Specimen. The procedure is essentially the same as for red blood cell counts, but employs a special diluting fluid.

Normal Range. 200,000 to 500,000 per cubic mm.

Red Cell Count

The red cells (erythrocytes) contain hemoglobin, the essential oxygen carrier of the blood. An increase in red cells may indicate hemoconcentration (insufficient water in the blood), or polycythemia, which is a condition characterized by a persistently elevated red cell count. A reduction in the red cells may come from hemorrhage or one of the anemias.

Procedure for Performing Test and Collecting Specimen. The finger or ear lobe is punctured and blood drawn into a special red cell pipette, up to a given mark. Diluting solution is then added to a second mark and the contents thoroughly mixed. The diluted suspension is then allowed to flow into a space in a special counting chamber. Using a microscope, the cells per unit area are then counted and the number of cells calculated.

Normal Range. 4,000,000 to 6,000,000 per cubic mm. (Note that the unit of volume used, a cubic mm., is only 1/1,000 of a cc.)

Reticulocyte Count

This test gives some indication of bone marrow activity. Reticulocytes are immature red blood cells. They retain a network of reticular material which can be stained with the proper dyes. When the bone marrow cells are very active, (a situation which occurs after hemorrhage and with recovery from anemia), there is an increase in the number of reticulocytes in the blood. When the bone marrow cells are less active, the number of reticulocytes in the blood falls. This test is often performed to evaluate the response to anemia therapy.

Procedure for Performing Test and Collecting Specimen. A thin film of cresyl blue is allowed to dry on a glass slide. A fresh drop of blood is then spread over the stain and kept moist to allow the stain to penetrate the cells. Using a microscope, the number of reticulocytes per 1,000 red blood cells is determined.

Normal Range. 0.1 to 4.0 reticulocytes per 100 red blood cells.

White Cell Count

White blood cells (leucocytes) are important in the defense of the body against invading microorganisms, since they destroy most harmful bacteria. An increase in the count is usually seen in infections. It may also be observed in other conditions including emotional upsets, blood disorders, and anesthesia. A decrease in the white blood cells may be seen in blood dyscrasias, overwhelming infections, and drug and chemical toxicity.

Procedure for Performing Test and Collecting Specimen. Essentially the same as for the red blood cell count, but a different pipette is used and a special diluting solution to hemolyze the red cells.

Normal Range. 4000 to 11,000 per cubic mm.

White Cell Differential Count

There are several kinds of white blood cells (leucocytes) which can be identified microscopically. It is often helpful to know whether the proportions of these cells in the blood have changed, in as much as that may direct attention to a particular group of diseases. The neutrophiles (neutral staining multinucleated cells) are increased in most bacterial infections. The eosinophiles (acid staining multinucleated cells) are increased in parasitic infestations and allergic conditions. The basophiles (basic staining multinucleated cells) may be increased in some blood dyscrasias. The lymphocytes may be increased in measles and in several bacterial infections. The monocytes may be increased during recovery from severe infections, Hodgkin's disease, and lipoid storage diseases. The reasons for these changes are not known.

Procedure for Performing Test and Collecting Specimen. A drop of fresh blood is placed on a slide and, using a second slide, is spread evenly over the surface of the glass in a thin film. After the film has dried, it is stained and examined under the microscope. Each type of white blood cell is counted separately. A total of 100 white cells of all kinds is counted, and the relative percentage of each calculated.

Normal Range:		
	Neutrophiles	54% to 62%
	Eosinophiles (acidophiles)	1% to 3%
	Basophiles	0% to 1%
	Lymphocytes	25% to 33%
	Monocytes	0% to 9%

Blood Types

Blood typing tests are important in patients who may need blood transfusions and in pregnant women. There are four main blood types, A, B, AB, and O, and several minor types. The letters refer to the kind of agglutinogen present in the red blood cells. Type A blood has A agglutinogen, B has B agglutinogen, AB has both A and B agglutinogen, and O has no agglutinogen. Each person has in his *serum* the agglutinins which react with all types of *agglutinogen not present* in his own cells. Thus A blood has anti-B agglutinin, B blood has anti-A agglutinin, AB has *no* agglutinin, and O has both anti-A and anti-B agglutinins. Whenever agglutinins in sufficient concentration come in contact with the corresponding agglutinogen, agglutination (clumping) of the red cells occurs, followed by rapid destruction of these cells. This often causes death. Thus if A blood is mixed with B or O type in equal amounts, the anti-A agglutinins in the other blood will clump and destroy the A cells. In most cases of incompatible transfusion, it is the *donor's* cells which are agglutinated by the recipient's (patient's) serum, rather than the reverse. The reason for this is that in a transfusion 500 cc. of donor's blood are added to approximately 5000 cc. of recipient's blood. The donor's blood is, therefore, diluted approximately 10 times. This weakens the agglutinins of the donor's blood so that ordinarily they cannot agglutinate red cells. However, the agglutinins of the recipient's blood are only diluted by 10 *per cent,* and remain strong. The dilution of the donor's blood does not affect the agglutinogens of the donor's red cells. Thus, the agglutinins of the recipient will clump the red cells of the donor in most incompatible transfusions. Exceptions occur only in those cases in which the donor has an unusually high concentration of agglutinins in his serum (high titer). In these rare cases the donor's agglutinins are powerful enough to remain active even after a 1:10 dilution and will clump the recipient's red cells.

It is usually advisable to transfuse only with the same type of blood as that of the recipient. However, in emergencies, type O blood (universal donor) is sometimes given to patients with different blood types. In most cases this is safe because the O cells of the donor have no agglutinogens and cannot be clumped by the recipient's serum. Also the 1:10 dilution of the donor's serum usually prevents it from clumping the recipient's red cells. There is, however, always the danger that the donor's serum may have a high agglutinin titer and clump the patient's blood. Therefore, when type O blood is given to patients of a different blood type, it is done as a calculated risk. In these cases constant observation of the patient is essential throughout the *entire* transfusion so that it may be stopped at once if a reaction occurs.

In a similar fashion the AB blood is called "universal recipient" and can usually receive blood of any type. Here, too, if the titer of the agglutinins in the donor's blood is high, a severe or even fatal reaction may occur. The same considerations and precautions that apply to the use of "universal donor" blood also apply, therefore, to "universal recipients" receiving blood of different types.

In recent years additional blood types have been found and probably more will be discovered. These other types exist in conjunction with the main groups and the Rh groups. Their importance is much less, although they have theoretical interest and are sometimes used with the other groups in cases of disputed paternity.

Rh Factor

The Rh factor is found in conjunction with any one of the main blood types. A person may be ARh+, ARh—, BRh+, BRh—, etc. The presence of the Rh factor is designated Rh+, its absence Rh—. The same considerations which apply to the main groups also apply to the Rh groups in transfusions. The Rh groups differ from the main blood groups in two important respects. First, the serum of an Rh— person does not ordinarily have significant amounts of anti-Rh agglutinins, unless there has been previous exposure to Rh+ blood. The previous exposure may have been a transfusion or injection of Rh+ blood, or pregnancy with an Rh+ fetus. With exposure to Rh+ blood, the Rh— person gradually builds up a high titer of anti-Rh agglutinins. The second difference between the Rh and main blood groupings is that in some cases anti-Rh agglutinin readily crosses the placental barrier, while the main agglutinins apparently do not do so in significant quantities. The importance of these aspects of the Rh factor lies not only in the area of blood transfusions, but also in pregnancy. The occurrence of erythroblastosis fetalis (destruction of the infant's red cells) in Rh+ babies born to Rh— mothers is commonly known and greatly exaggerated. Because of the need for prior exposure to Rh+ blood before large amounts of anti-Rh agglutinins are produced, the first Rh+ child of an Rh— mother will almost always be normal unless the mother has had a transfusion or injection of Rh+ blood. Also, many Rh— women have several normal Rh+ children, since there is considerable variation in the titer of anti-Rh agglutinin produced by different individuals and also in the amounts of anti-Rh agglutinin which pass the placental barrier.

Procedure for Collecting Specimen. Venous blood is

withdrawn and 5 cc. placed in a test tube and allowed to clot.

Laboratory Procedure. There are several methods of typing blood, each with its own advantages and disadvantages. In general, all methods depend on the mixing of the patient's red cells with separate standard serum samples of groups A and B. As an additional check, the patient's serum is mixed with red cell suspensions of A and also of B types. The type of serum which agglutinates the patient's red cells and the type of red cell agglutinated by the patient's serum indicate the patient's blood type. A similar test is used to distinguish between Rh– and Rh+ blood. False positive as well as false negative reactions can occur, so that these tests are entrusted to a skilled and experienced person. A mistake in blood typing may be responsible for the death of the patient.

Blood Urea Nitrogen (B.U.N.) —*See Urea Nitrogen*

Blood Urea Nitrogen (B.U.N.)

This is a sensitive test for liver function. When Bromsulphalein is injected intravenously, about 80 per cent of it is removed by the liver and about 20 per cent by other organs. If the liver does not function properly, a larger amount than normal of the injected Bromsulphalein will remain in the blood. If marked jaundice is present, the test cannot be performed satisfactorily and is not needed.

There have been reports of serious and fatal sensitivity reactions to Bromsulphalein. *Therefore, it is recommended that on the injection tray there be an extra syringe and needle, and an ampul of epinephrine.*

Procedure for Collecting Specimen. The patient cannot receive any other dyes for 2 days before the test, and must be fasting for 12 hours. He is weighed just before the test and 5 mg. of Bromsulphalein dye per kg. of body weight is injected intravenously by the physician. It is essential that none of the dye be allowed to leak into the tissues, since it is highly irritant and causes sloughing. After exactly 45 minutes have passed, 5 cc. of venous blood is withdrawn from the opposite arm, placed in a test tube, and allowed to coagulate. The test is performed on the serum.

Laboratory Procedure. The amount of Bromsulphalein in the serum sample is determined colorimetrically. Marked jaundice will make the measurements unsatisfactory.

Normal Range. Less than 0.4 mg. of Bromsulphalein per 100 cc. of serum.

B.S.P. —*See Bromsulphalein Retention*

B.U.N. —*See Urea Nitrogen*

Calcium

Calcium is one of the essential ions in the body. It is needed for many vital processes such as muscular contraction, nerve transmission, and blood clotting. The minimum concentration of calcium ions required for each of these processes differs somewhat. Only ionized calcium is effective, and unfortunately there is no satisfactory method of measuring ionized calcium levels. However, the total amount of calcium, ionized and nonionized, can be determined. It is generally believed that about 50 per cent of the total calcium is ionized. If there is any acidosis, the percentage of ionized calcium is higher. In alkalosis, the percentage of ionized calcium is lower. The total calcium level alone does not indicate the amount of ionized calcium.

When there is a deficiency in ionized calcium, the major manifestation is a generalized tetanic condition beginning with twitching of muscle fibers and finally producing tetanic convulsions. This condition is probably due to the response of the nerves or neuromuscular junctions to the reduced calcium levels. It is unlikely that blood clotting changes are related to calcium levels, since normal clotting can take place at calcium levels considerably lower than those which would be fatal because of the production of severe, sustained tetanic convulsions. Therefore, calcium determinations are of no value in disorders of blood clotting.

A decrease in the blood calcium, called hypocalcemia, occurs in several conditions. In celiac disease and sprue, absorption of calcium from the gastrointestinal tract is impaired. In hypoparathyroidism, the balance between blood calcium and bone calcium is disturbed, and in some kidney diseases excess calcium is lost in the urine.

An increase in the blood calcium (hypercalcemia) is found in a number of conditions, including hyperparathyroidism (overfunctioning of the parathyroids), multiple myeloma, and respiratory diseases with increased carbon dioxide tension (concentration) in the blood.

Procedure for Collecting Specimen. Venous blood is withdrawn and 6 cc. placed in a test tube and allowed to coagulate. The test is performed on the serum.

Laboratory Procedure. Two methods are generally in use. The chemical method involves the precipitation of calcium as the oxalate, followed by titration with potassium permanganate. Calcium levels may also be determined by flame photometry where suitable apparatus is available.

Normal Range. 9.0 to 11.5 mg. per 100 cc. of serum, or 4.5 to 5.8 milliequivalents per liter.

Carbon Monoxide

In suspected carbon monoxide poisoning, the identification of significant amounts of carbon monoxide in the blood establishes the diagnosis. The test is not restricted to acute carbon monoxide poisoning which frequently has a fatal outcome before the doctor arrives. There are many cases of chronic, low grade carbon monoxide poisoning causing such symptoms as headache, malaise and weakness. They are not easily diagnosed except by determination of the blood carbon monoxide level and usually result from occupational exposure to exhaust gases in industrial plants, garages, etc. They may also come from defective gas-burning appliances in the home. Most persons have small amounts of carbon monoxide in their blood from exposure to tobacco smoke, automobile exhaust fumes, etc.

Procedure for Collecting Specimen. Venous blood is withdrawn and 5 cc. placed in a bottle with oxalate. The usual method is quantitative estimation by means of a spectrograph.

Normal Range. Less than 0.8 volume per cent of blood.

Cephalin Flocculation

This test is useful in diagnosing liver damage. The serum of normal persons, properly diluted, will not flocculate (clump) a colloidal suspension of cephalin and cholesterol. On the other hand, the serum of persons whose liver cells are damaged does flocculate the suspension. This test is sensitive and frequently positive in the early stages of liver disease before jaundice appears. It is negative in acute obstruction of the biliary tract of short duration. If the obstruction persists, secondary damage to the liver cells occurs and the cephalin flocculation test becomes positive. Certain types of liver disease which do not damage the liver cells give a negative reaction, for example, neoplasms and abscesses. Some nonhepatic disorders, such as malaria, kala-azar, and rheumatoid arthritis, may sometimes produce a positive reaction. A positive test, therefore, is not of itself conclusive. Since this test affords a rough quantitative measurement of liver cell function, it is sometimes used to follow the course of patients with a known liver disease, such as cirrhosis. The results are reported as negative to 4+.

Procedure for Collecting Specimen. Venous blood is withdrawn and 5 cc. placed in a test tube and allowed to coagulate. The test is performed on the serum.

Laboratory Procedure. A 1:20 dilution of the serum is added to a suspension of cephalin and cholesterol. The extent of flocculation is observed at the end of 24 and 48 hours.

Normal Range. Either negative or 1+. Reports are delayed 24 to 48 hours.

Chlorides

Chlorides are measured to help diagnose disorders in the maintenance of normal osmotic relationships, acid-base balance, and water balance of the body. Usually this test is performed together with measurement of other ions of the blood.

An elevation in blood chlorides (hyperchloremia) occurs in several conditions, including various kidney disorders, Cushing's syndrome, and hyperventilation. A decrease in blood chlorides (hypochloremia) is seen in such states as excessive vomiting and diarrhea, diabetic acidosis, Addison's disease, heat exhaustion, and following certain surgical procedures.

Procedure for Collecting Specimen. Venous blood is withdrawn and 5 cc. placed in a test tube and allowed to clot. The test is performed on the serum.

Laboratory Procedure. The chlorides are precipitated by silver iodate, leaving a soluble iodate which is titrated with sodium thiosulfate.

Normal Range. This may be expressed in various ways: 100 to 106 milliequivalents per liter of serum, or 355 to 376 mg. of chloride per 100 cc. of serum, or 585 to 620 mg. of *sodium chloride* per 100 cc. of serum or plasma.

Cholesterol

Cholesterol is a normal constituent of the blood and is found in all cells but its exact physiologic function is not clear. It may serve as the substance from which various hormones are synthesized. In various disease states the cholesterol concentration in the serum may be raised or lowered. Cholesterol levels are elevated in many conditions; in most the finding is only incidental. An elevated cholesterol level may be helpful in the diagnosis of xanthomatosis, certain liver diseases, and hypothyroidism. There is also increasing interest in the role of cholesterol in producing myocardial infarction since deposits of cholesterol, known as plaques, are often found partially blocking the coronary arteries. However, there is as yet no conclusive evidence linking this condition to the blood serum cholesterol concentration. Decreased serum cholesterol is found in hyperthyroidism, anemias, starvation, and acute infections.

Procedure for Collecting Specimen. Venous blood is withdrawn and 5 cc. placed in a test tube and allowed to coagulate. The test is performed on the serum.

Laboratory Procedure. Total cholesterol is hydrolyzed with alkali and precipitated with digitonin. The precipitate is redissolved and reagents added which produce a color. The color intensity, measured with a colorimeter, is proportional to the concentration. This test usually takes about 48 hours.

Normal Range. 120 to 260 mg. per 100 cc. of serum.

Cholesterol Esters

In addition to free cholesterol, there are cholesterol esters in the serum. Their physiologic role is unknown. The proportion of cholesterol esters is normal in some xanthomatoses. The proportion of esters is low in some obstructions of the common bile duct, but the total amount is normal. In cases where liver cells are damaged, there is a drop in both absolute and relative amounts of the esters. The determination of the esters may therefore be helpful in assessing the amount of cellular damage in the liver.

Procedure for Collecting Specimen. Venous blood is withdrawn and 7 cc. placed in a test tube and allowed to coagulate. The test is performed on the serum.

Laboratory Procedure. Total cholesterol is measured as described above. On another sample, the free cholesterol is determined by following the same procedure but omitting hydrolysis with alkali. The difference between free and total cholesterol values represents the quantity of cholesterol esters. This test usually requires about one week.

Normal Range. 68 to 78 per cent of the total cholesterol.

Clotting (Coagulation) Time

This test measures the ability of blood to clot. Many factors are involved in clotting, including prothrombin, thromboplastin, and fibrinogen. New clotting factors are continually being discovered. A deficiency of any essential factor or an increase in inhibitory factors may prolong clotting time. This test is distinct from the bleeding time test since the latter also involves the ability of small blood vessels to constrict. This test, furthermore, should not be confused with special clotting time measurements that use siliconized or lusteroid test tubes.

Procedure for Performing Test and Collecting Specimen. There are several methods. The most common ones involve the use of venous blood. Freshly drawn blood is put into 4 small test tubes (1 cc. in each) and the first tube is tilted at 30-second intervals. When clotting is observed, the same procedure is followed in succession with the other 3 tubes. The clotting time is the average of the times elapsed between venipuncture and clotting in the last 3 tubes.

Normal Range. 10 to 25 minutes *by this method.* Using other methods of measurement, normal clotting time may may be 1 to 5 minutes.

Coagulation

See Clotting Time

CO_2 Combining Power

This test, sometimes referred to as CO_2 capacity, is a general measure of the acidity or alkalinity of the blood.

An increase in CO_2 combining power is usually a manifestation of alkalosis, while a decrease is usually a manifestation of acidosis. However, changes in CO_2 combining power do not always represent changes in pH of the blood, since the latter depends on the ratio, not on the absolute amounts, of basic and acidic substances. As in many other tests, good clinical judgment is needed to evaluate the results. High CO_2 combining power is usually found in conditions such as persistent vomiting or drainage of the stomach with loss of hydrochloric acid, excessive intake of sodium bicarbonate in the presence of poor kidney function, excessive administration of ACTH or cortisone, and hypoventilation. Low CO_2 combining power is usually found in such conditions as diabetic acidosis, severe diarrhea or drainage of intestinal fluids, certain kidney diseases, and hyperventilation. In many cases it is also necessary to test the pH of the blood to evaluate properly the acid-base balance. The CO_2 combining power test may, in some situations, be designated by the physician as "emergency."

Procedure for Collecting Specimen. Venous blood is withdrawn and 8 cc. carefully placed in a test tube containing oil. Excessive contact of the blood with air may give incorrect results. When blood for several tests is drawn into a single syringe, it is advisable first to fill those containers which require oil.

Laboratory Procedure. Usually the Van Slyke apparatus is used. The serum sample is equilibrated with alveolar air. Then the carbon dioxide, combined with the serum, is freed by adding an acid and the volume measured.

Normal Range. 56 to 70 volumes per 100 cc. of serum, or 25 to 31 millimols per liter of serum.

Congo Red Retention

This is a test for amyloidosis. In this disease deposits of amyloid tissue are laid down in such organs as liver, kidneys and spleen, and eventually interfere with proper function. The amyloid material has an affinity for Congo red and removes it from the blood. In patients with amyloid disease, therefore, the dye disappears from the blood more rapidly than in normal humans. In advanced amyloidosis 60 to 99 per cent of the dye may be removed in 4 minutes. The test may be negative in the early stages of the disease. In albuminuria associated with hypoproteinemia there may be a false positive reaction.

Procedure for Performing Test and Collecting Specimen. At least 2 days must elapse between the injection of any other dye, such as B.S.P., and this test. The physician injects intravenously 0.3 cc. of a 1% solution of Congo red per kg. of body weight, completing the injection within 1 minute. Exactly 5 minutes later, 6 cc. of venous blood is drawn from the opposite arm and placed in a test tube, where it coagulates. Exactly 1 hour after the injection of the dye another 6 cc. sample of venous blood is drawn and placed in another test tube. After the second blood sample has been collected, a specimen of urine is also obtained.

Laboratory Procedure. The amount of dye in the serum is determined colorimetrically.

Normal Range. Less than 40 per cent of the injected dye disappears from the blood in 1 hour.

C-Reactive Protein (C.R.P.)

The C-reactive protein test is a test for inflammation and tissue breakdown. Thus it is non-specific and similar to the sedimentation rate test (Page 81). The C-reactive protein test is positive in myocardial infarction, acute rheumatic fever, widespread cancers, bacterial infections and other conditions. It is sometimes used to follow the activity of a disease. The term C-reactive protein was chosen because the protein involved forms a precipitate with the C-polysaccharide of the pneumococcus. The relationship between this action and its use in diagnosis is not clear, and the clinical use of the test is based on the empirical observation that it is positive in conditions with widespread inflammation and tissue breakdown.

Procedure for Collecting Specimen. There are two separate procedures in use. If the test is to be performed in the laboratory, clotted blood is needed. Venous blood is withdrawn and 5 cc. placed in a test tube and allowed to coagulate. The test is performed on the serum.

If the test is to be performed at the bedside, a fingertip technique may be used. Special capillary tubes are used, and capillary blood is drawn into the tube and allowed to clot. After standing, the clot is discarded, leaving the serum for the test.

Laboratory Procedure. A sample of the serum is mixed with C-reactive protein antiserum. If a precipitate forms, the test is positive.

Normal Range. No C-reactive protein present.

Creatinine

This test is a measurement of kidney function similar to the urea nitrogen test. Creatinine is derived from the breakdown of muscle creatine phosphate. The amount produced per day is relatively constant, and it is excreted by the kidney. An elevated blood creatinine level indicates a disorder of kidney function.

Procedure for Collecting Specimen. Venous blood is withdrawn and 6 cc. placed in a test tube and allowed to coagulate. The test is performed on the serum.

Laboratory Procedure. To the serum sample is added alkaline picrate. The color produced is compared to standards and the concentration of creatinine calculated.

Normal Range. 0.6 to 1.3 mg. per 100 cc. of serum.

Differential Count

See Blood Counts, White Cell Differential Count

Fasting Blood Sugar (F.B.S.)

See Glucose (Sugar)

Fibrinogen

In conditions characterized by inadequate blood clotting it may be helpful to determine which element of the clotting mechanism is deficient. The fibrinogen of the plasma is essential for blood clotting. In the presence of thrombin it is converted to insoluble fibrin threads. Measurement of the blood fibrinogen level may aid in establishing the cause of a clotting deficiency.

Procedure for Collecting Specimen. Venous blood is withdrawn and 5 cc. placed in a bottle with oxalate. The test is performed on the plasma.

Laboratory Procedure. To the sample of plasma is added sodium sulfite which precipitates the fibrinogen. The amount of fibrinogen is measured by the biuret test.

Normal Range. 200 to 600 mg. per 100 cc. of plasma. Plasma normally contains more fibrinogen than is actually needed for satisfactory clotting. Deficiencies in blood clotting due to fibrinogen deficiency do not occur until the concentration falls to 75 mg. per 100 cc. of plasma.

Globulin

See Albumin, Globulin, Total Protein, A/G Ratio

Glucose (Sugar)

This test is performed to discover whether there is a disorder of glucose metabolism. An increase in blood glucose level is found in severe diabetes, chronic liver disease, and overactivity of several of the endocrine glands. A symptom caused directly by the elevated blood sugar is occasional, intermittent blurring of vision. In mild diabetes there may be a normal glucose level, so that more sensitive tests need to be performed (see *Glucose*

Tolerance). There may be a decrease in blood sugar in tumors of the islets of Langerhans in the pancreas, underfunctioning of various endocrine glands, glycogen storage disease (von Gierke's), and overtreatment with insulin. If the blood glucose level falls too low, coma, convulsions, and even death may result.

Procedure for Collecting Specimen. Venous blood is withdrawn and 3 to 5 cc. placed in an oxalate bottle.

Laboratory Procedure. After precipitation of proteins the glucose in the filtrate is oxidized with cupric or ferricyanide solution. The amount present is then determined colorimetrically.

Normal Range. 70 to 105 mg. per 100 cc. of serum, or 60 to 90 mg. per 100 cc. of whole blood.

Glucose Tolerance

These tests are used to discover disorders of glucose metabolism which have not become severe enough to change the blood glucose levels in the fasting state. In the glucose tolerance tests, a large amount of glucose is given to a fasting patient, either intravenously or orally. At regular intervals thereafter, the blood glucose levels are measured to learn how long it takes the body to handle the added glucose. If it remains in the blood for an excessive period of time, there is some disorder of carbohydrate metabolism. The intravenous test is somewhat more sensitive than the oral, since the factor of absorption from the gastrointestinal tract is not involved. In the oral test, an increase in blood sugar and its persistence for 3 hours is seen in diabetes. In the intravenous test the blood sugar is, of course, elevated in all cases. If the blood glucose concentration does not return to normal within less than 3 hours after the intravenous administration of glucose, diabetes is probably present. If 1 to 2 hours are required to return to normal there may be some liver disorder. The urine voided during the course of this test is examined for sugar to obtain additional information about the kidney excretion of excess sugar.

Procedure for Collecting Specimen. The patient must have been on an adequate diet for at least 3 days before the test and must have fasted for the preceding 12 hours. The following steps are taken in order:

1. Withdraw venous blood and place 3 cc. in an oxalate or fluoride bottle supplied by the laboratory.
2. Collect urine specimen at once.
3. If the intravenous test is used the doctor will administer intravenously by slow infusion 0.5 Gm. of glucose per kg. of body weight. He will use a 20% solution and take 30 minutes for the infusion.

3a. If the oral test is used, the patient receives 1.75 Gm. of glucose per kg. of body weight in unsweetened lemonade.

4. If the intravenous test is used, 3 cc. of venous blood is withdrawn immediately from the arm which did not receive the infusion; subsequent withdrawals are made exactly 30, 60, 90 and 150 minutes following the infusion. The blood is

placed in an oxalate or fluoride bottle. With each sample, a urine specimen is collected.

4a. In the oral test, 3 cc. of venous blood is collected 30, 60, 120 and 180 minutes after ingestion of the glucose and placed in an oxalate bottle. With each blood sample a urine specimen is also collected.

5. Each specimen must be labeled with the date and time of collection.

Laboratory Procedure. The laboratory will test each blood sample as described under *Glucose* and each urine sample as described under *Sugar, Qualitative, Chapter 5.*

Normal Range. Oral: Peak of not more than 150 mg. per 100 cc. of serum; return to fasting level within 2 hours. Intravenous: Return to fasting level within about 1 hour.

Grouping

See Blood Types

Hematocrit

This test measures the relative volume of cells and plasma in the blood. In anemias and after hemorrhage the hematocrit reading is lowered; in polycythemia and dehydration it is raised.

Procedure for Collecting Specimen. Venous blood is withdrawn and 4 cc. placed in an oxalate bottle.

Laboratory Procedure. The oxalated blood is carefully placed in a special (Wintrobe) tube up to the 0 mark.

The tube is then spun in a centrifuge and the height of the column of packed red blood cells measured against the gradations on the side of the tube.

Normal Range. For women, 35 to 45 mm. of red blood cells per 100 mm. of column height; for men, 40 to 50 mm.

Hemoglobin

Hemoglobin, the essential oxygen carrier of the blood, is found within the red blood cells and is responsible for the red color of the blood. The hemoglobin is decreased in hemorrhage and anemias and increased in hemoconcentration and polycythemia. The hemoglobin and red cell count do not always rise or fall equally. This fact is often important in differential diagnosis of anemias. In iron deficiency (microcytic) anemia, hemoglobin is reduced more than the red blood cell count. In pernicious anemia, the red cell count is reduced more than hemoglobin.

Procedure for Performing Test and Collecting Specimen. Capillary blood is employed.

A commonly used procedure is the Sahli method. The finger or ear lobe is punctured and blood drawn into a special pipette up to a mark. The blood is then placed in a special graduated test tube and diluted hydrochloric acid added, converting the hemoglobin to acid hematin. The mixture is then diluted util it matches the color of a standard. The amount of hemoglobin is determined by measuring the height of the fluid column against the graduations on the side of the test tube.

Normal Range. 12 to 18 Gm. per 100 cc. of blood.

Heterophile Antibody

This is a test for infectious mononucleosis. In this disease the level of antibodies to sheep erythrocytes rises for reasons that are not known. If the titer rises above a specified level, the test is considered probably positive. However, sometimes there are other anti-sheep erythrocyte antibodies in the blood, which are not related to infectious mononucleosis. Accordingly, it may be necessary to repeat the test by using more complicated techniques of antibody absorption.

Procedure for Collecting Specimen. Venous blood is withdrawn, and 5 cc. placed in a test tube and allowed to coagulate. The test is performed on the serum.

Laboratory Procedure. Serial dilutions of the patient's serum are added to washed suspensions of sheep erythrocytes in a series of test tubes and incubated. The greatest dilution which agglutinates the erythrocytes is noted.

Normal Range. Agglutination in concentrations up to 1:28.

Icterus Index

This is a measure of the degree of yellowness of the serum. It is a simple way to determine whether there is excess bilirubin (bile pigment) in the serum. The test, however, cannot differentiate between bilirubin due to excess hemolysis, or that due to obstruction of the biliary tract. The test is useful in discovering early jaundice not yet visible, or in following the course of frank jaundice.

Procedure for Collecting Specimen. Venous blood is withdrawn and 5 cc. placed in a test tube and allowed to clot. This test is performed on the serum.

Laboratory Procedure. The color of the serum is compared to the color of a standard solution of potassium bichromate, using a colorimeter.

Normal Range. 4 to 6 units.

Insulin Tolerance

This test is useful in differentiating between hypopituitarism and primary hypothyroidism. After injection of insulin in the former condition, the blood glucose level drops to about 50% in 20 to 30 minutes. In the latter condition, the fall is less and requires at least 45 minutes. This test is of no value in the diagnosis of hyperinsulinism.

Procedure for Collecting Specimen. The patient must have been on an adequate diet for 3 days and have fasted for 12 hours before the test. *Before proceeding with the test there must be on hand a concentrated glucose solution in a sterile syringe.* This may be a life-saving precaution.

A sample of venous blood is withdrawn and 3 cc. placed in a fluoride bottle. The doctor injects the insulin intravenously. Ordinarily the dose is 0.1 unit of regular insulin per kg. of body weight. However, if Addison's disease or adrenal insufficiency is suspected, the dose is less: 0.03 unit per kg. of body weight.

The patient is watched *continuously* for a possible sudden reaction. A physician should be on the floor to treat any severe reaction immediately with intravenous glucose. A reaction often begins with extreme nervousness, hunger, sweating and salivation. Disorders of speech and vision occur, and tremors and convulsions may be seen.

Venous blood samples (3 cc.) are collected 20, 30, 45, 60, 90 and 120 minutes after administration of insulin and placed in fluoride bottles. Care must be taken to label each blood sample with time of collection.

Laboratory Procedure. Same as described under *Glucose.*

Normal Range. A return to the pre-injection level within 2 hours.

L.E.

See Lupus Erythematosus Cell Test

Lipase

This is a test for damage to the pancreas. Like amylase, lipase is secreted by the pancreas, and small amounts pass into the blood. In diseases such as acute pancreatitis and carcinoma of the pancreas, the blood level of lipase rises.

Both amylase and lipase levels rise at the same rate, but the elevation in lipase concentration persists for a longer period. The lipase determination is, therefore, made when too much time has elapsed for the amylase level to remain elevated.

Procedure for Collecting Specimen. Venous blood is withdrawn and 6 cc. placed in a test tube and allowed to coagulate. The test is performed on the serum.

Laboratory Procedure. The serum sample is incubated with emulsified tributyrin. The amount of butyric acid liberated is titrated.

Normal Range. Not over 1.5 units.

Lupus Erythematosus (L.E.) Cell Test

A particular type of leucocyte, called the lupus erythematosus cell, is often seen in lupus erythematosus. Finding this cell can help in the diagnosis, although it may also be found in other conditions.

Procedure for Collecting Specimen. Venous blood is withdrawn and 5 cc. placed in an oxalate bottle.

Laboratory Procedure. The leucocytes of the blood are concentrated by centrifugation, smeared and stained. The stained smears are then examined microscopically.

Normal Range. Normally there are no lupus erythematosus cells.

Malaria Film

This is a test for malaria parasites in the blood. It is important not only in establishing a definite diagnosis of malaria but also in determining which species of malarial parasite is involved. Each species can be identified on the film.

Procedure for Performing Test and Collecting Specimen. A film of blood is placed on a slide and stained with Giemsa stain. Depending on the number of parasites, a thin or thick film of blood may be best. The slides are examined microscopically for parasites.

Normal Range. Normally there are no malaria parasites in the blood.

Methemoglobin

Methemoglobin is not ordinarily present in the blood. It is found when the hemoglobin is oxidized by chemicals such as nitrites, chlorates, etc. Drinking well water containing nitrites is a frequent cause of methemoglobinemia. Methemoglobin is not an oxygen carrier like hemoglobin.

Procedure for Collecting Specimen. Venous blood is withdrawn and 5 cc. placed in an oxalate bottle.

Laboratory Procedure. Methemoglobin is detected by the use of the spectroscope which shows the absorption bands of this substance when light is passed through it.

Normal Range. Normally there is no methemoglobin in the blood.

Non-Protein Nitrogen (N.P.N.)

This is a general test of kidney function. It is not as sensitive as certain other tests and cannot be used to discover early kidney disease. About half of the non-protein nitrogen is usually urea, which is normally excreted by the kidney. The remainder consists of amino acids, ammonia, creatine, creatinine, uric acid, and some unidentified substances. When kidney function is markedly diminished, the urea, and, therefore, the non-protein nitrogen level in the blood, rises. This measurement is less accurate than the urea nitrogen test.

Procedure for Collecting Specimen. Venous blood is collected and 5 cc. placed in an oxalate bottle.

Laboratory Procedure. The nitrogenous substances are converted to ammonia which is then measured by titration.

Normal Range. 15 to 35 mg. per 100 cc. of serum.

P.B.I.

See Protein-Bound Iodine

pH

This is a measure of acidity or alkalinity. The normal blood pH ranges from 7.35 to 7.45. The pH may be lower in such conditions as hypoventilation, severe diarrhea, Addison's disease, and diabetic acidosis. The pH may rise above normal levels in conditions such as excess vomiting, Cushing's syndrome, and hyperventilation.

Procedure for Collecting Specimen. Venous blood is withdrawn and 5 cc. placed in a test tube under a layer of oil. The test is performed on the serum.

Laboratory Procedure. A sensitive pH-meter measures the pH electronically.

Normal Range. pH 7.35 to 7.45.

Phosphatase, Acid

This is a test to determine metastasizing carcinomas of the prostate. Normally, small amounts of acid phosphatase are found in the serum. The prostate gland is exceptionally rich in this enzyme and so are carcinomas of the prostate. The normal gland and the carcinoma which has not yet spread do not release the enzyme into the serum. However, the metastasizing prostate carcinoma does, increasing the serum concentration markedly. The test is performed only on men.

Procedure for Collecting Specimen. Venous blood is removed and 2.5 cc. placed in each of 2 test tubes (total 5 cc.) and allowed to clot. The test is performed on the serum.

Laboratory Procedure. The speed with which a sample of serum hydrolyzes a monophosphate ester at pH 5 is measured.

Normal Range. Up to 2.5 King-Armstrong units, or up to 1.5 phenol units.

Phosphatase, Alkaline

This test may be used in the diagnosis of bone as well as of liver diseases. Normally, there is a small amount of alkaline phosphatase in the serum. In bone diseases, however, the alkaline phosphatase rises in proportion to the formation of new bone cells. This test, therefore, may be of value in differentiating between various bone disorders, including tumors. In disorders of the liver and biliary tract, the alkaline phosphatase rises because excretion is impaired. This test may therefore also be of some use in evaluating the degree of blockage of the biliary tract.

Procedure for Collecting Specimen. Venous blood is withdrawn and 2.5 cc. placed in each of 2 test tubes (total 5 cc.) and allowed to clot. The test is performed on the serum.

Laboratory Procedure. The speed with which a sample of serum hydrolyzes a phosphate ester at pH 9.7 is measured.

Normal Range. Adults, 1.5 to 4 Bodansky units; children, up to 20 Bodansky units.

Phosphorus

Phosphorus metabolism is directly associated with calcium metabolism and involves many organs and physiological functions. The concentration of phosphorus may be increased in severe kidney disease, hypoparathyroidism, acromegaly, or excessive vitamin D intake. The concentration may decrease in rickets, hyperparathyroidism, and certain diseases of the kidney tubules.

Procedure for Collecting Specimen. Venous blood is withdrawn and 4 cc. placed in a test tube and allowed to coagulate. The test is performed on the serum.

Laboratory Procedure. A protein-free sample of the serum is added to the standard reagents which produce a blue color. The intensity of the color is then measured with a colorimeter.

Normal Range. Adults, 3.0 to 4.5 mg. per 100 cc. of serum; children, 4 to 6.5 mg. per 100 cc. of serum.

Platelet Count

See Blood Counts, Platelet Count

Potassium

Potassium is an essential ion found in large concentrations in all cells and in much smaller concentrations in the serum. Alterations in serum potassium levels may produce serious changes in body function, or even death. A marked decrease in serum potassium may cause cardiac arrhythmias and muscle weakness; a marked increase produces a series of electrocardiographic changes and arrhythmias. There may also be depression, lethargy, and coma. Therefore, when it is suspected that serum potassium levels have changed, tests should be made and measures taken to restore them to the normal range. Increased serum potassium levels may be found in conditions of severe cell damage and destruction, adrenal cortical deficiency, and hypoventilation. A decrease in serum potassium may be found in severe diarrhea, periodic familial paralysis, chronic kidney disease, excess function of the adrenal cortex, and following administration of insulin and glucose in diabetes without added potassium. Low serum potassium levels are particularly dangerous when digitalis glycosides are being administered.

Procedure for Collecting Specimen. Venous blood is withdrawn, preferably with a special oiled syringe and 6 cc. placed in a test tube under oil. The oil is used to minimize friction and the resulting hemolysis of red cells.

Laboratory Procedure. The serum concentration of potassium is measured in a flame photometer.

Normal Range. 4 to 5 milliequivalents per liter or 16 to 22 mg. per 100 cc. of serum.

Protein-Bound Iodine (P.B.I.)

This is a test of thyroid function. The thyroid gland binds iodine to organic compounds, mainly the hormone thyroxin. This hormone is precipitated by chemicals which precipitate proteins, so that a measurement of the amount of iodine in a protein precipitate indicates the amount of thyroid hormone present. An increased concentration of protein-bound iodine is usually found in hyperthyroidism, although it may also be seen in early hepatitis. A decreased concentration of protein-bound iodine is usually found in hypothyroidism.

Procedure for Collecting Specimen. The patient must not have been given any radio-opaque, iodine-containing material for procedures such as intravenous pyelography or cholecystography during the preceding six months period. He should not have received thyroid hormones for the preceding 14 days. Venous blood is withdrawn and 8 cc. placed in a test tube and allowed to coagulate. The test is performed on the serum.

Laboratory Procedure. A protein precipitant is added to a sample of serum and the precipitate removed, washed, treated with alkali, and redissolved. Its ability to decolorize a yellow solution of ceric sulfate indicates the iodine content.

Normal Range. 3.0 to 8.0 microgm. per 100 cc. of serum.

Protein, Total

See Albumin, Globulin, Total Protein, A/G Ratio

Prothrombin Time

This is an indirect test of the clotting ability of the blood. Prothrombin is converted to thrombin in the clotting process. When the prothrombin level of the blood is lower than normal, it is believed that the clotting tendency of the blood within the blood vessels is diminished. The prothrombin content of the blood is lowered in liver diseases, hypoprothrombinemia of infants, vitamin K deficiency, and following drug therapy. The vast majority of cases of low blood prothrombin results from the administration of Dicumarol or similar drugs. These substances are given to reduce the clotting tendency of the blood and thus avoid thromboembolic phenomena.

Procedure for Collecting Specimen. The patient need not be in a fasting state. Venous blood is withdrawn and exactly 4.5 cc. placed in a special test tube containing a special sodium oxalate solution, and mixed thoroughly. Ordinary oxalate bottles cannot be used.

Laboratory Procedure. There are several methods. The most commonly used is the one-stage method of Quick where a mixture of thromboplastin and calcium is added to the oxalated serum. The time of formation of fibrin threads is measured with a stop-watch. This result is then compared to that obtained on normal blood.

Normal Range. Between 11 and 18 seconds, depending on type of thromboplastin used, is considered 100 per cent of normal. In Dicumarol treatment the physician tries to keep the prothrombin time at 2 to 2½ times normal. Expressed as prothrombin percentage, which is not a straight-line function of prothrombin time, a range of from 20 to 30 per cent is sought.

Red Cell Count

See Blood Counts, Red Cell Count

Red Cell Fragility

This is a test of the ability of the red blood cells to resist hemolysis in a hypotonic solution. As the concentration of salts outside the cell decreases, more water continues to pass into the cell by osmosis, and the membrane finally bursts. The salt concentration at which hemolysis occurs is taken as a measure of red blood cell fragility. Fragility is increased in congenital hemolytic jaundice and aplastic anemia.

Procedure for Collecting Specimen. Venous blood is withdrawn into a completely dry syringe and 5 cc. placed in an oxalate bottle. For control purposes a similar 5 cc. sample is drawn from a normal person and placed in another oxalate bottle labeled "control."

Laboratory Procedure. Samples of the blood are added to solutions of sodium chloride varying in concentration from 0.28% to 0.6%, by steps of 0.02%. After gentle mixing, the mixtures are allowed to stand for several hours. The presence of hemolysis is shown by a clear red coloration of the supernatant plasma.

Normal Range. Slight hemolysis between 0.40% and 0.46% sodium chloride; complete hemolysis between 0.30% and 0.36% sodium chloride.

Reticulocyte Count

See Blood Counts, Reticulocyte Count

Rh Factor

See Blood Types, Rh Factor

Sedimentation Rate

This test measures the rate at which red cells settle to the bottom of a glass test tube. The sedimentation rate is increased in infections and in conditions in which cell destruction occurs. This test is useful in diagnosing and following the course of such illnesses as rheumatic fever, arthritis and myocardial infarction.

Procedure for Collecting Specimen. Venous blood is withdrawn and 4 cc. placed in an oxalate bottle.

Laboratory Procedure. A sample of the blood is placed in a special thin glass tube which is kept upright. The rate at which the upper part of the red cell column descends is measured and is usually reported as millimeters fall in 1 hour. Corrections for anemia are sometimes made and reported as "corrected" sedimentation rate.

Normal Range. This depends to some extent on the type of glass tube used. In the Westergren method, which is common, the normal values for men are 0 to 15 mm. per hour and for women 0 to 20 mm. per hour.

Serological Tests (General)

These tests are used to identify substances in the serum which result from exposure to certain microorganisms. Often, the substance to be identified and quantitated is an antibody to the microorganism itself. An example is the Widal test for typhoid antibodies. Sometimes, the material of interest is an antibody to some enzyme elaborated by a microorganism, for example, antistreptolysin O. In many cases, however, the exact relationship between the microorganism and the serological material is unknown. Years of observation have shown that, in the presence of a particular disease, the body elaborates a substance which is readily measured. For example, in infectious mononucleosis, the body produces larger amounts than usual of antibodies to sheep red blood cells (see *Heterophile Antibody*). Similarly, we do not understand the relationship of the serological tests for syphilis to the Treponema which causes the disease.

Procedure for Collecting Specimen. Venous blood is withdrawn and 5 cc. placed in a test tube and allowed to coagulate. The test is performed on the serum.

Laboratory Procedure. This varies with the type of test.

Normal Range. There may be weak positive reactions to some serological tests in the absence of disease.

Serological Tests for Syphilis

There are several varieties, including the Wassermann, Kolmer, Kahn and Mazzini test. All are non-specific in nature and sometimes they are positive in diseases other than syphilis. Interpretation of these serological tests usually requires considerable skill and experience, as well as correlation with the clinical findings and history. In early primary syphilis the serology is negative. In late, adequately treated syphilis, the serology may be fixed at a high positive titer although the patient is, in effect, cured. In late, improperly treated syphilis, the serology may be negative even though the patient is not cured and is developing central nervous system involvement.

Serological tests for syphilis are performed routinely in many situations, often because of legal requirements. For example, many states require a serological test before marriage. Most physicians have these tests performed on all pregnant women to avoid congenital syphilis in the newborn. Many hospitals require a routine serology on all patients on admission.

Procedure for Collecting Specimen. Venous blood is withdrawn and 5 cc. placed in a test tube and allowed to coagulate. The test is performed on the serum.

Laboratory Procedure. This varies with the test being performed.

Normal Range. Normally these tests are negative. If the reaction is faintly positive, it may denote some disorder other than syphilis.

Serum Albumin . . . Serum Globulin . . . Serum Protein

See Albumin, Globulin, Total Protein, A/G Ratio

Serum Transaminase

This test is used primarily in the diagnosis of myocardial infarction, to distinguish it from acute coronary insufficiency without infarction.

Transaminases are enzymes which catalyze the transfer of an amino grouping (NH_2) from an amino acid to an alpha keto acid. There are several different kinds of transaminases. The most commonly measured one is the glutamic oxaloacetic transaminase (sometimes abbreviated GOT). Transaminases are found normally in heart, liver, muscle, kidney and pancreas. Elevated serum levels are seen in myocardial infarction, viral hepatitis and other liver diseases.

In myocardial infarction, transaminase levels are 4 to 10 times normal and remain high up to 5 days. In liver disease, they may be 10 to 100 times normal. There are moderate elevations in other diseases at times. Thus it should be clear that there is nothing specific in transaminase levels, and that their value in diagnosis depends on careful comparison with the results of physical examinations and other laboratory tests.

Procedure for Collecting Specimen. Venous blood is withdrawn and 5 cc. placed in a test tube and allowed to coagulate. The test is performed on the serum.

Laboratory Procedure. There are several methods for determining transaminase. Currently, both colorimetric and spectrophotometric measurements are in common use.

Normal Level. 40 units.

Sickle Cell Test

This test is performed to demonstrate an unusual type of red blood cell, containing a different type of hemoglobin which is relatively insoluble when unoxygenated. When the available oxygen is reduced the hemoglobin may precipitate within the cell, causing it to assume the shape of a sickle. This may interfere with the free flow of blood and cause various disorders. Most people with the sickling trait in their red cells have no demonstrable disease but may require special care and attention in surgery and obstetrics to avoid hypoxia (diminution of oxygen supply). Although the sickling trait is more often found in Negroes, it may also be found in other persons.

Procedure for Performing Test and Collecting Specimen. There are several methods; the simplest employs a solution of sodium bisulfite in water. A drop of the solution is added to a drop of blood and the blood examined microscopically for the sickle-shaped cells.

Normal Range. Sickling is not a disease in the usual sense. There is no normal or abnormal range.

Sodium

Sodium is the main cation of the blood and extracellular fluid. Its concentration may vary within narrow limits, but if these are exceeded, serious disturbances or even death may result. Increased serum sodium levels may be found in markedly inadequate water intake and following administration of excessive amounts of sodium. Decreased sodium levels may occur in diarrhea, heat exhaustion, Addison's disease and certain kidney disorders.

Procedure for Collecting Specimen. Venous blood is withdrawn, preferably with a special oiled syringe and

6 cc. placed in a test tube under oil. The oil is used to minimize friction and the resulting hemolysis of red blood cells.

Laboratory Procedure. The serum concentration of sodium is measured in a flame photometer.

Normal Range. 138 to 145 milliequivalents per liter or 315 to 335 mg. per 100 cc. of serum.

Sugar

See Glucose

Sulfhemoglobin

Sulfhemoglobin is not ordinarily found in the blood. It is produced when sulfides combine with the hemoglobin in the blood. It is usually associated with the intake of excessive amounts of acetanilid or phenacetin.

Procedure for Collecting Specimen. Venous blood is withdrawn and 5 cc. placed in an oxalate bottle.

Laboratory Procedure. The blood is examined spectroscopically for the absorption bands in the transmitted light beam.

Normal Range. Normally there is no sulfhemoglobin in the blood.

Sulfonamide Level

In treating patients with sulfonamide drugs it is often helpful to know the concentration of the drug in the blood in order to decide whether to change dosage. This test measures the concentration of sulfonamides in the blood and may be adapted to measure their concentration in any body fluid.

Procedure for Collecting Specimen. Venous blood is withdrawn and 5 cc. placed in an oxalate bottle.

Laboratory Procedure. A protein-free sample of serum is mixed with a reagent which gives a red color. The intensity of the color is measured in a colorimeter.

Normal Range. Normally there are no sulfonamides in the blood. The therapeutic level sought varies not only with the specific drug used but also with the invading microorganism. Some bacteria are much more sensitive to sulfonamides than others. In general, levels of between 5 and 15 mg. per 100 cc. of serum are sought.

Thymol Turbidity

This is a test of liver function. Normally, when serum is mixed with a saturated solution of thymol, turbidity is seen. The turbidity is usually increased in liver conditions, such as hepatitis, where the liver cells are damaged. In biliary obstruction without damage to the liver cells the turbidity is usually normal.

Procedure for Collecting Specimen. Venous blood is withdrawn and 5 cc. placed in a test tube and allowed to coagulate. The test is performed on the serum.

Laboratory Procedure. A sample of serum is added to a saturated solution of thymol. The degree of turbidity produced is measured colorimetrically or by comparison with a set of standards.

Normal Range. Less than 5 units.

Total Cholesterol

See Cholesterol

Total Protein

See Albumin, Globulin, Total Protein, A/G Ratio

Urea Clearance

See Urea Clearance, Chapter 5

Urea Nitrogen (Blood Urea Nitrogen)

This is a test of kidney function. Ordinarily the kidney readily excretes urea, the end-product of protein metabolism, so that the blood urea concentration is fairly low. However, in certain kidney disorders the ability to excrete urea may be impaired, so that the concentration of urea nitrogen in the blood increases. This test gives essentially the same information as the non-protein nitrogen (N.P.N.) test and is somewhat more accurate. There is no reason to do both tests and in most hospitals one or the other is performed. A rising blood urea nitrogen level may portend mental clouding, confusion and disorientation, and the patient may eventually go into coma. Therefore, when the laboratory report indicates a rising blood urea nitrogen content, the nurse should be prepared to deal with a patient who might become difficult to handle.

Procedure for Collecting Specimen. Venous blood is withdrawn and 5 cc. placed in an oxalate bottle.

Laboratory Procedure. The urea is converted to ammonia by the enzyme urease. The amount of ammonia is then measured by titration with acid.

Normal Range. 9 to 17 mg. of urea nitrogen per 100 cc. of blood The amount of actual urea, as distinct from urea nitrogen, ranges from 19 to 36 mg. per 100 cc. of blood but this value is seldom mentioned clinically.

Uric Acid

This test is usually performed to diagnose gout but it may also give significant results in other conditions. Uric acid is the end-product of purine metabolism and purines come mainly from cell nuclei. The blood uric acid concentration in gout is high. The reason for this is unknown. The uric acid concentration may also be elevated in conditions involving marked cellular destruction such as leukemia, pneumonia and toxemias of pregnancy. With severe kidney damage there may be an elevated uric acid level because of decreased excretion. However, this does not afford an accurate index of kidney function.

Procedure for Collecting Specimen. Venous blood is withdrawn and 5 cc. placed in an oxalate bottle.

Laboratory Procedure. A sample of serum is added to a reagent or mixture of reagents which produce a blue color with uric acid. The intensity of the color is measured and the concentration of uric acid calculated.

Normal Range. 3.5 to 6 mg. per 100 cc. of serum.

Van den Bergh Test

See Bilirubin, Partition

White Cell Count

See Blood Counts, White Cell Count

White Cell Differential Count

See Blood Counts, White Cell Differential Count

4

Tests Performed on Cerebrospinal Fluid (C.S.F.)

Cerebrospinal fluid, often called spinal fluid, fills the ventricles of the brain and the central canal of the spinal cord. It acts as a fluid buffer which can enlarge or diminish in volume, when necessary, to protect the brain and spinal cord from compression injury when slight changes occur in the volume of the space enclosed by the cranium and spinal column. It may also help prevent traumatic jarring of the brain. The cerebrospinal fluid may also play a role in supplying oxygen and nutrients to the brain and cord and removing waste.

Cerebrospinal fluid is produced from blood by the choroid plexus, a highly vascular structure in the brain ventricles. It differs from a filtrate of blood in several respects, and the exact mechanism by which it is formed is not known. It is, however, in osmotic equilibrium with the blood.

From the brain ventricles where it is produced, the cerebrospinal fluid passes slowly down the spinal canal and is slowly reabsorbed into the blood. Approximately 100 cc. of cerebrospinal fluid is normally present and usually that amount is produced and reabsorbed daily.

Because of its intimate association with the brain and spinal cord, cerebrospinal fluid is a useful indicator of disease in those organs.

Usually, cerebrospinal fluid is obtained by lumbar puncture. In this procedure the physician withdraws fluid after passing a needle between two lumbar vertebrae into the spinal canal. Lumbar puncture is to be viewed as the equivalent of a surgical operation. The same sterile precautions are essential. In some institutions the patient must sign a permission form before lumbar puncture can be performed.

In a few cases the cerebrospinal fluid is obtained by puncture of the cisterna magna. This requires insertion of a needle between the base of the skull and the first cervical vertebra. It can be done safely by physicians specially trained in this technique.

After the needle has entered the spinal canal the physician usually performs several tests of the cerebrospinal fluid pressure. Only after these have been done are fluid samples withdrawn for laboratory examination. The fluid samples are not placed in a single container, but into a series of small test tubes, usually 3 or 4, depending on the tests ordered. The test tubes must be kept in the correct order, since the first tubes are more likely to contain minute amounts of blood from the puncture. Those tests which would be affected by small amounts of blood are therefore performed on fluid contained in the last tubes.

Cell Count

This test often indicates the presence of infection, such as meningitis. It is usually performed immediately following lumbar puncture and requires only about 15 minutes. The cell count is moderately increased (10 to 200 per cubic millimeter) in such conditions as poliomyelitis, encephalitis and neurosyphilis. Cell counts of several thousand per cubic millimeter are found in most cases of meningitis.

Procedure for Collecting Specimen. The physician places 1 to 2 cc. of cerebrospinal fluid in a special small test tube. Usually the third tube in the series is used, since it is less likely to contain minute amounts of blood.

Laboratory Procedure. The diluting fluid is drawn up to the first mark in the white cell pipette (used in white blood cell counts) and the spinal fluid is then drawn up to another mark. After mixing, a part of the mixture is placed in a counting chamber and the white cells counted with the aid of a microscope.

Normal Range. 0 to 8 cells per cubic millimeter.

Chlorides

The cerebrospinal fluid chlorides are reduced in some types of meningitis, particularly tuberculous meningitis. Measurement of the chloride level may aid in differential diagnosis.

Procedure for Collecting Specimen. The physician places 2 cc. of cerebrospinal fluid in a special small test tube.

Laboratory Procedure. The same as for blood chlorides.

Normal Range. 720 to 760 mg. of sodium chloride per 100 cc. of spinal fluid. Note that this value is usually given in terms of mg. of sodium chloride per 100 cc., while the concentration of chlorides in serum is usually expressed as milliequivalents of chloride per liter.

Colloidal Gold

This test is performed to help diagnose diseases of the central nervous system. It is nonspecific, and positive results may be obtained not only in neurosyphilis but also in meningitis, multiple sclerosis, poliomyelitis, encephalitis and other serious disorders of the central nervous system. The test depends on alterations of albumin-globulin ratios in the spinal fluid. Normal spinal fluid does not precipitate colloidal gold, whereas abnormal fluid does.

Procedure for Collecting Specimen. The physician places 1 cc. of cerebrospinal fluid in a special small test tube. Bloody spinal fluid will give a false positive reaction and cannot be used.

Laboratory Procedure. Samples of the spinal fluid, diluted with different concentrations of saline, are placed in 10 test tubes in order of decreasing saline concentration. Colloidal gold suspension is added to each and the mixture allowed to stand over night. The extent of precipitation in each test tube gives a pattern which suggests a particular disease.

Normal Range. Either no precipitation of the colloidal gold, or 1+ precipitation in a few test tubes.

Culture

See Spinal Fluid Culture, Chapter 2

Protein

The spinal fluid protein is increased in several diseases of the central nervous system, especially meningitis and subarachnoid hemorrhage. Qualitative tests are now being replaced with simple quantitative tests of greater accuracy.

Procedure for Collecting Specimen. The physician places 2 cc. of cerebrospinal fluid in a special small test tube. The last test tube of cerebrospinal fluid collected should be used for protein determination.

Laboratory Procedure. To the sample of cerebrospinal fluid is added sulfosalicylic acid which precipitates the protein. The degree of precipitation indicates approximately the amount of protein present.

Normal Range. 15 to 40 mg. per 100 cc. of spinal fluid.

Serological Tests

These tests are performed to discover the presence of neurosyphilis. A positive serological reaction of the spinal fluid almost always indicates neurosyphilis.

Procedure for Collecting Specimen. The physician places 7 cc. of spinal fluid in a small test tube.

Laboratory Procedure. A Wassermann test is performed which is similar to that done on the blood.

Normal Range. Normally the serological reaction is negative.

Sugar

Spinal fluid sugar is decreased in meningitis. This test is often useful in the differential diagnosis of central nervous system conditions.

Procedure for Collecting Specimen. The physician places 2 cc. of cerebrospinal fluid in a special small test tube. If the test cannot be performed at once, breakdown of sugar must be prevented by preservation with a thymol crystal.

Laboratory Procedure. The Folin-Wu method is usually employed. This involves the use of specially shaped test tubes. The degree to which the spinal fluid sample changes the color of cuprous oxide in the presence of molybdate-phosphate is compared to controls in a colorimeter.

Normal Range. 50 to 80 mg. per 100 cc.

5

Tests Performed on Urine

Urine is formed by the kidneys. The glomeruli of the kidneys allow a filtrate of the blood plasma to pass into the tubules. The cells lining the tubules selectively reabsorb most of the filtrate. The tubule cells may also excrete certain substances into the urine being formed. During a 24-hour period a total of about 200 liters of fluid is filtered through the glomeruli and about 199 liters are reabsorbed by the tubules. The difference represents the urine excreted.

Although it is believed that the primary function of the kidneys is excretion of wastes, other functions are as important if not more so. They include regulation of ionic balance, acid-base balance and water balance of the body. Urine will vary widely in composition from time to time and such variations are indicative of good function and are not abnormal.

Some authorities divide tests of kidney function into three groups: those which test glomerular filtration (e.g., urea clearance), those which test tubular reabsorption (e.g., concentration and dilution tests), and those which test the excretion by the tubules (e.g., phenolsulfonphthalein excretion tests). Many kidney disorders, however, may involve both glomeruli and tubules, so that interpretation of the results of these tests requires considerable skill and experience. There are also many tests of urine which are done to evaluate the condition of organs other than the kidney.

Aceto-Acetic Acid

See Diacetic Acid

Acetone

This test is important in the diagnosis of ketosis, a type of acidosis produced by faulty metabolism. In a condition such as diabetes, sugar is not utilized properly and excessive fat is metabolized. The fatty acids are broken down into aceto-acetic acid and B-hydroxybutyric acid. These cannot be completely disposed of by the tissues in the presence of impaired carbohydrate metabolism. They are converted to acetone which is then excreted by the kidneys. Acetone in the urine indicates a severe disorder of metabolism. The patient may exhibit symptoms of depression of the central nervous system.

Procedure for Collecting Specimen. A urine sample is placed in a bottle and sent to the laboratory.

Laboratory Procedure. To the urine sample are added ammonium sulfate and a nitroprusside solution. Ammonia is then layered on top. A red to purple ring forms at the interface of the two layers if acetone is present.

Normal Range. Normally there is no acetone in the urine.

Addis Test

This is a method for determining the kind of kidney disease present. The number of cells and casts in the urine sediment are counted. A comparison of the amounts of each suggests the type of kidney disorder.

Procedure for Collecting Specimen. If the patient is known to have severe renal disease with such signs as elevation of the urea nitrogen, this test should not be performed. For 24 hours all fluids, including coffee and soup, are stopped. The diet is otherwise normal. After approximately 12 hours without fluid, the patient urinates and the specimen is discarded. The time of voiding is noted. For the next 12 hours all urine specimens are voided directly into a large, clean, dry bottle and the total specimen collected. In some institutions female patients are catheterized; in others they are allowed to void into the bottle after washing and drying the vulva. The bottle is kept sealed and in a cool place until the end of the test, when it is delivered to the laboratory.

Laboratory Procedure. The entire specimen is mixed thoroughly. Then a sample of urine is centrifuged and the sediment examined microscopically. The number of white blood cells, red blood cells and casts are counted, and the total number of each excreted in the 12-hour period is calculated.

Normal Range: Per 12-hour specimen:
Red blood cells–0 to 450,000
White blood cells–30,000 to 1,000,000
Hyaline casts–0 to 5,000

Albumin, Qualitative

Ordinarily the albumin in the blood does not pass through the glomerular wall into the urine. However, in several conditions such as kidney disease, hypertension, severe heart failure or drug toxicity, albumin appears in the urine. It may also be seen in orthostatic albuminuria which is not a disease. Therefore, the test is not specifi- but indicates that more precise tests are needed.

Procedure for Collecting Specimen. A urine specimen is placed in a bottle and sent to the laboratory.

Laboratory Procedure. A sample of urine is boiled in a test tube. When a cloud appears, glacial acetic acid is added. Persistence of the cloud indicates albumin. The results are reported as negative, or 1+ to 4+, depending on the density of the cloud.

Normal Range. In 5 to 15 per cent of normal individuals small amounts of albumin are sometimes found in the urine with no disease present. This has been termed orthostatic or postural albuminuria.

Albumin, Quantitative

This test is performed to discover the amount of albumin lost daily in the urine. This information may be helpful in attempting to restore protein balance.

Procedure for Collecting Specimen. The urine excreted during a 24-hour period is collected in a clean bottle and sent to the laboratory.

Laboratory Procedure. Several methods may be used. They involve the addition of reagents which precipitate the albumin. The amount of precipitate or degree of turbidity is then compared to standards.

Normal Range. Normally there is no albumin in the urine.

Aschheim-Zondek Test

This is a test for pregnancy. During pregnancy hormones are produced and excreted in the urine. When the urine of a pregnant woman is injected into immature animals, these hormones can stimulate the animal's ovaries, so that they simulate early pregnancy in the animal. A quantitative Aschheim-Zondek test is sometimes performed to diagnose teratoma and chorionepithelioma (malignant tumors).

Procedure for Collecting Specimen. About 75 cc. of morning urine is placed in a bottle and sent to the laboratory.

Laboratory Procedure. Small amounts of urine are injected into immature female mice daily for 3 days. On the fifth day the animals are killed and the ovaries examined. If there are hemorrhagic follicles, the test is positive.

Normal Range. In the absence of pregnancy this test is negative.

Ascorbic Acid (Vitamin C) Tolerance

This test measures the degree of vitamin C deficiency. When a large dose of the vitamin is given intravenously in normal persons, about 30 per cent or even more will be excreted in the urine. In deficiency states, much less will be excreted.

Procedure for Collecting Specimen. The patient must be on a diet free of ascorbic acid for 24 hours before the test. The bladder is emptied and the urine discarded. The physician then administers 1 Gm. of ascorbic acid in 10 cc. of saline intravenously. All urine voided during the next 24 hours, including a specimen voided at the end of 24 hours, is collected in a brown urine bottle which is kept in a refrigerator. The patient may have water during the test. In some institutions the test is conducted over a period of less than 24 hours.

Laboratory Procedure. The amount of ascorbic acid in the urine is measured by its ability to decolorize a solution made blue by the addition of a special reagent.

Normal Range. About 30 per cent of the amount administered is excreted.

Bence-Jones Protein

This is a test for bone tumors. Bence-Jones protein is an unusual type of protein molecule with a molecular weight of about 35,000 as compared to 70,000 for albumin. it coagulates on heating at about 45° C. and redissolves at about 100° C. It is excreted in large amounts in the urine in most cases of multiple myeloma. It may also be found in other types of bone tumors.

Procedure for Collecting Specimen. A urine sample is placed in a bottle and sent to the laboratory.

Laboratory Procedure. The urine sample is acidified to pH 5 and heated to 45° to 70° C. If coagulation of protein is seen, the urine is heated to 100° C. If the coagulum is due to Bence-Jones protein, it redissolves at 100° C. and recoagulates at 70° C. or less.

Normal Range. Normally there is no Bence-Jones protein in the urine.

Bile and Bilirubin

This is a test of liver function. Bile pigments and acids are found in the urine when there is obstruction of the biliary tract. Bilirubin (the main pigment) is found alone when there is excessive hemolysis of the red blood cells.

Procedure for Collecting Specimen. A urine specimen is placed in a bottle and sent to the laboratory. The test for bile acids cannot be performed if the urine specimen has been preserved with thymol.

Laboratory Procedure. The test for bilirubin is performed by layering concentrated nitric acid on the urine sample in a test tube. Many colors at the junction of the liquids indicate bilirubin. The test for bile acids is performed by sprinkling some finely powdered sulfur on the surface of the cold urine. The speed with which the sulfur sinks indicates roughly the amount of bile acids present.

Normal Range. Normally bile acids and bilirubin are not found in the urine.

Blood

Blood in the urine may appear as intact red blood cells (hematuria) or dissolved hemoglobin derived from destroyed red blood cells (hemoglobinuria). Hematuria comes from bleeding somewhere along the urinary tract from glomerulus to urethra. The site of bleeding and its cause are determined by more precise testing methods. Hemoglobinuria usually arises from conditions outside the urinary tract. The red cells are hemolyzed and the dissolved hemoglobin in the plasma is excreted by the kidney. It is seen in severe burns, transfusion reactions, severe malaria (blackwater fever), poisoning, and paroxysmal hemoglobinuria.

Procedure for Collecting Specimen. A urine specimen is placed in a bottle and sent to the laboratory.

Laboratory Procedure. Intact red blood cells are identified by centrifuging the urine and examining the sediment microscopically. Hemoglobin is identified either by guaiac or benzidine tests. Either of these produces a blue color if hemoglobin is present.

Normal Range. In the male there is normally no blood in the urine. In the female, blood, due to menstrual flow, may be found. A catheterized specimen may contain blood because of urethral bleeding from the trauma of inserting the catheter.

Calcium Test (Sulkowitch)

This test measures roughly the amount of calcium in the urine. In hypoparathyroidism the urinary excretion of calcium is decreased. This test is therefore useful in cases of tetany to determine quickly whether the cause is hypoparathyroidism.

Procedure for Collecting Specimen. A urine sample is placed in a bottle and sent to the laboratory.

Laboratory Procedure. To a sample of urine is added an equal volume of Sulkowitch reagent. The extent of precipitation indicates roughly the amount of calcium. Absence of a precipitate indicates an abnormally low serum calcium.

Normal Range. A fine white precipitate indicates a normal concentration of serum calcium.

Chlorides, Quantitative

This examination is performed to evaluate the urinary excretion of chlorides. It is useful in the management of cardiac patients on low salt diets and in adjusting fluid and ion balance in postoperative cases.

Procedure for Collecting Specimen. The total urine excreted over a 24-hour period is collected in a large bottle.

Laboratory Procedure. A simplified test, using a manufactured tablet, is now replacing the more complex analytical chemical techniques.

Normal Range. This may vary considerably with salt intake and with perspiration. In general, most of the ingested chloride, less that lost in perspiration, is excreted in the urine. Thus there is really no "normal" or "abnormal" range and the values obtained in this test are significant only in relation to the balance between intake and output. Usually there are about 9 Gm. of sodium chloride per liter of urine.

Concentration and Dilution

These tests measure the ability of the kidneys to concentrate and dilute urine, an indication of their functional capacity. Inadequate concentration or dilution of urine indicates some disorder of the tubules of the kidneys.

Procedure for Collecting Specimen. The procedures vary in different institutions. A fairly common one is the following:

First night:

1. At supper the patient is restricted to 1 glass of fluid.
2. Thereafter no food or drink is given until the end of the test.
3. The patient remains in bed as much as possible.
4. Before going to sleep the patient empties the bladder and the urine is discarded.
5. On arising the patient passes a urine specimen which is saved.
6. Second and third specimens are collected 1 and 2 hours later. The exact time of voiding each specimen is recorded.
7. After the third specimen the patient may have food and drink.

Second night:

8. A regular supper is eaten.
9. No food or drink is allowed thereafter, except as specified.
10. The patient is kept in bed as much as possible.

11. On awakening in the morning, the patient empties the bladder and the urine specimen is discarded.
12. After urination the patient is given 5 glasses of fluid to drink within 45 minutes. The fluid may be water, lemonade or weak tea.
13. Urine is collected 1, 2, 3 and 4 hours after the patient has started drinking.
14. After the 4-hour specimen has been collected, the patient may have food and drink.

Laboratory Procedure. The specific gravity of each urine specimen is measured with a urinometer.

Normal Range. For concentration phase, specific gravity of 1.026 or over. For dilution phase, specific gravity of about 1.003 in first urine specimen, gradually increasing thereafter.

Diacetic (Aceto-Acetic) Acid

This test is used in the diagnosis of metabolic ketosis. Like acetone, diacetic acid is produced when glucose is not properly utilized, and excessive fat is metabolized. A positive test for diacetic acid indicates a more severe degree of ketosis (acidosis) than a positive acetone test alone. The patient may develop weakness, headache, thirst, air hunger, epigastric pain and vomiting. These symptoms may progress to restlessness and confusion or to symptoms of central nervous system depression. If untreated, coma and death may ensue.

Procedure for Collecting Specimen. A urine sample is placed in a bottle and sent to the laboratory.

Laboratory Procedure. To a sample of urine in a test tube is added a 10% solution of ferric chloride. A purple color indicates diacetic acid. Certain coal tar breakdown products may give a false positive test.

Normal Range. Normally there is no diacetic acid in the urine.

Fermentation Test for Sugar

This test differentiates between the various kinds of sugar in the urine. Not all sugar found in the urine is glucose. Other sugars which may be present are fructose, galactose, lactose, and various pentoses (sugars with 5 carbons). The presence of these sugars does not indicate diabetes, but usually means there is some other metabolic defect. It may be important in some cases to make sure whether or not the sugar found in the urine is glucose.

Procedure for Collecting Specimen. A urine sample is placed in a bottle and sent to the laboratory.

Laboratory Producedure. The urine sample, to which yeast is added, is placed in a special fermentation tube and kept in an incubator for a period of time. If glucose is present, carbon dioxide will be produced through fermentation and will be readily visible because of the shape of the container.

Normal Range. Normally there is no sugar in the urine.

Friedman Test

This is a test for pregnancy and is basically the same as the Aschheim-Zondek, but employs a female rabbit.

Glucose Tolerance —*See Glucose Tolerance, Chapter 3*

17-ketosteroid Excretion

The 17-ketosteroids are male hormones with a ketone group on the 17th carbon atom of the phenanthrene ring. In men two-thirds of these hormones are produced by the adrenals and only one-third by the testes. In women virtually all of these materials are secreted by the adrenals. Accordingly, it should be clear that, although they are male hormones, the level of 17-ketosteroid excretion is usually more important in diagnosing disorders of the adrenals than disorders of the testes.

In children the level of 17-ketosteroids is normally very low. Low levels of these compounds are found in adrenal hypofunction from any cause, including Addison's disease, myxedema, pituitary hypofunction and many types of severe debilitating illness.

High levels of 17-ketosteroids are found in certain types of adrenal or testicular hyperfunction. In women with virilizing syndromes, the 17-ketosteroid excretion is usually moderately elevated.

Very marked elevations, over 100 mgm. a day, suggest either carcinoma of the adrenal cortex or the extremely rare interstitial cell tumor of the testis.

Procedure for Collecting Specimen. Into a large bottle, usually of gallon size, 3 cc. of acetic acid is placed as a preservative. The patient's urine for a 24-hour period is then collected in this bottle. If the patient has been receiving bicarbonate of soda, a greater amount of acetic acid might be required to maintain the acidity of the specimen.

Laboratory Procedure. One method in common use is the measurement, colorimetrically, of the intensity of a red color produced when M-dinitrobenzene is added.

Normal Range. Adult males, 8 to 20 mgm. per day; adult females, 5 to 15 mgm. per day.

Lead

In suspected lead poisoning the determination of lead concentration in the urine may aid in diagnosis.

Procedure for Collecting Specimen. The patient must be on a low calcium diet for at least 3 days before the test to mobilize the lead from the bones. Collect a 24-hour specimen in a special large bottle.

Laboratory Procedure. Both chemical and spectrographic methods are available. The latter method is preferred and is based on the absorption of specific wavelengths of light by the lead.

Normal Range. 0.020 to 0.080 mg. per liter of urine.

Melanin

This test is an aid in the diagnosis of melanoma. Melanin or its precursor, melanogen, appears in the urine in this disease but is also found in several other conditions.

Melanin colors the urine brown or black. Melanogen is colorless.

Procedure for Collecting Specimen. A urine sample is placed in a bottle and sent to the laboratory.

Laboratory Procedure. To a sample of urine is added sodium nitroprusside and sodium hydroxide. If a deep red color appears, glacial acetic acid is added and the instant production of a blue color indicates melanogen.

Normal Range. Normally there is no melanin or melanogen in the urine.

Melanogen

See Melanin

Microscopic Tests

Microscopic examination of the urinary sediment may reveal important information about the condition of the urinary tract. Red blood cells in males, or in females who are not of menstrual age, suggest bleeding somewhere along the tract, from glomerulus to urethra. When red blood cells are found, further studies are usually performed to determine the exact source of the blood. White blood cells (pus cells) in males or in catheterized specimens from females suggest infection of the urinary tract. Casts in the urine suggest some disorder of the kidney tubules. Crystals of certain kinds (sulfonamide) may indicate a need for change in therapeutic regimen.

Procedure for Collecting Specimen. A urine specimen is placed in a bottle and sent to the laboratory.

Laboratory Procedure. A sample of the urine is centrifuged and the sediment examined microscopically.

Normal Range. Normally there are no red blood cells and very few pus cells in the urine of males. In females of menstrual age, they may be found unless a specimen collected by careful catheterization is sent for examination. A few casts may be found normally, but large numbers of casts suggest kidney disease.

Oral d-Xylose Tolerance Test

This is a test of the ability of the gastrointestinal tract to absorb nutrients. There are several disorders of absorption which, if accurately diagnosed, can be corrected by appropriate treatment.

The d-xylose is ordinarily absorbed by the gastrointestinal tract and then excreted by the kidney. If, after ingestion, the amount found in the urine is low (assuming kidney function is adequate), it is probable that a disorder of gastrointestinal absorption exists. The d-xylose is used instead of glucose because several conditions may produce misleading absorption figures with glucose.

Procedure for Collecting Specimen. The patient must fast overnight. Urine is voided and discarded. Then, 25 Gm. of d-xylose are mixed with 500 cc. of water and swallowed. After one hour an additional 250 cc. of plain water is taken, and another hour later, another 250 cc. All urine is collected for 5 hours from the ingestion of the d-xylose. At least 150 cc. of urine must be voided and collected.

Laboratory Procedure. A sample of urine is heated with a special reagent mixture which changes the xylose into a pink-colored material. The intensity of the color is compared to a standard in a colorimeter.

Normal Range. 5 to 8 Gm. of d-xylose in the urine in 5 hours (20 to 32% absorption).

pH

This is a measure of the degree of acidity or alkalinity of the urine. The kidney maintains the blood at the correct pH by excreting into the urine any excess ions which might alter the pH of the blood. The urinary pH, therefore, varies widely and changes do not indicate abnormality. However, in certain situations it is advisable to have an acid or alkaline urine and the pH measurement is important. When sulfadiazine is administered or when there is marked hemolysis or destruction of muscle tissue (crush syndrome), an alkaline urine is needed to keep the excreted substances soluble. Sulfadiazine, and the products of hemolysis and muscle destruction, are quite soluble in an alkaline urine, but in acid urine they precipitate and may cause urinary blockage and death. In treatment with certain urinary tract antiseptics (methenamine) an acid urine is needed. In bladder infections the urine may be highly alkaline because bacteria transform urea into ammonia.

Procedure for Collecting Specimen. A urine specimen is placed in a bottle and sent to the laboratory. In infants treated with sulfadiazine, the urinary pH is important, but collection of a urine sample may be difficult. A simple expedient is to place a strip of nitrazine paper inside the diaper at each change. The pH of the urine is then determined by the color of the nitrazine paper at the next diaper change.

Laboratory Procedure. A strip of nitrazine paper is dipped into the urine. The color change, compared to a standard chart, indicates the pH.

Normal Range. pH 4.8 to 8.0.

Phenolsulfonphthalein (P.S.P.) Test

This is a test of the ability of the kidney tubules to excrete a dye. The urinary excretion of injected phenolsulfonphthalein is decreased in chronic nephritis and urinary tract obstructions. It may be increased in certain liver diseases.

Procedure for Collecting Specimen. The patient voids and the specimen is discarded. Then the patient drinks 2 glasses of water. Thirty minutes after the initial urine specimen is passed the physician injects 1 cc. of phenolsulfonphthalein solution intravenously. Urine specimens are then collected in separate containers at intervals of 15, 30, 60 and 120 minutes after injection of the dye and sent to the laboratory.

Laboratory Procedure. The urine samples are alkalinized to bring out the maximum color and compared to standards in a colorimeter.

Normal Range. Elimination of 63% to 84% of the

injected dye in 2 hours. For greater sensitivity the percentage excreted in each fraction is calculated.

Phenylketonuria Test

This test is designed to uncover early cases of phenylketonuria (phenylpyruvic oligophrenia). In this condition the patient—an infant—is unable to metabolize phenylalanine, an essential amino acid, properly. As a result, pathologic metabolic end-products are formed which lead to permanent mental deficiency. If the disorder is recognized early, a phenylalanine deficient diet can be given and the mental deficiency avoided. Accordingly, it is important to recognize the disorder as soon as possible. In some hospitals a routine diaper test is performed on all infants over 4 weeks of age, since infants with this disorder excrete phenylpyruvic acid in the urine after the age of 3 weeks.

Procedure for Collecting Specimen. Several pieces of absorbent or filter paper are placed in the baby's diaper by the mother or nurse. After they have been wet with urine, they are dried and sent to the laboratory.

Laboratory Procedure. A dried paper strip is tested with a drop of 10% ferric chloride solution. If phenylpyruvic acid is present the paper turns green, and the green color fades in 5 minutes. If the test is positive or doubtful, more precise chemical tests can be performed on the other papers for confirmation.

Normal Range. Normally there is no phenylpyruvic acid in the urine, and the test is negative.

Porphyrins

Porphyrins are pigments, similar to bilirubin, and probably come from the hemoglobin of the blood. Normally there is an insignificant amount of porphyrin in the urine. In certain conditions, such as toxic liver damage, lead poisoning, some blood disorders, pellagra, and congenital porphyria, the urinary excretion of porphyrins rises.

Procedure for Collecting Specimen. The total urine excreted by the patient over a 24-hour period is collected in a large bottle.

Laboratory Procedure. The urine is treated so as to precipitate and concentrate any porphyrins which may be present. The redissolved precipitate is examined spectroscopically for the absorption bands characteristic of porphyrins.

Normal Range. A minute quantity may normally be found in the urine.

P.S.P.

See Phenolsulfonphthalein Test

Routine Analysis

This comprises the tests for albumin, sugar, specific gravity, pH, and microscopic examinations. A single random urine specimen is used for all these examinations.

Specific Gravity

This measurement indicates the degree of concentration of dissolved material in the urine. Ordinarily the specific gravity rises when the fluid intake is low and falls when fluid intake is high. In certain kidney disorders involving the tubules the urine is not concentrated or diluted beyond relatively narrow limits.

Procedure for Collecting Specimen. A urine sample is placed in a bottle and sent to the laboratory.

Laboratory Procedure. The extent to which a standard urinometer sinks in the urine determines the specific gravity.

Normal Range. 1.001 to 1.030.

Sugar

See Fermentation Test for Sugar

Sugar, Qualitative

In some disorders sugar is found in the urine. This occurs most often in diabetes mellitus, but may also occur in other metabolic disorders of varying importance. Because of its simplicity this test is usually employed as a screening procedure to discover diabetes. If sugar is found, other tests may then be ordered to determine the type of sugar (see *Fermentation Test for Sugar*).

Procedure for Collecting Specimen. A urine sample is placed in a bottle and sent to the laboratory.

Laboratory Procedure. The more complex tests of a few years ago have now been replaced with simplified tablet tests. A specified amount of urine is added to a tablet and the color produced indicates the presence or absence of sugar.

Normal Range. Normally there is no sugar in the urine.

Sugar, Quantitative

This test is performed on some diabetics to determine the extent of sugar loss.

Procedure for Collecting Specimen. A 24-hour urine specimen is collected in a clean bottle and sent to the laboratory.

Laboratory Procedure. A sample of the urine is titrated with Benedict's quantitative solution. The disappearance of color from the Benedict's solution marks the end-point.

Normal Range. Normally there is no sugar in the urine.

Sulkowitch Test

See Calcium Test (Sulkowitch)

Urea Clearance

This is a test of function of the glomeruli of the kidneys. The ability of the kidneys to remove urea from the blood is measured and expressed in terms of volume of blood cleared of urea per minute. Urea clearance is decreased in kidney disease.

Procedure for Collecting Specimen. The patient may have a light breakfast before the test but cannot have coffee, tea, cocoa, or milk. During the test the patient remains in bed, arising only to void.

1. At the beginning of the test the patient is given 400 cc. of water to drink.
2. At the end of 30 minutes the patient empties his bladder completely and this urine specimen is discarded.
3. One and one-half hours after the beginning of the test the patient again empties his bladder completely into a clean, dry bottle. If necessary, 200 cc. of water may be given to help the patient empty his bladder. The exact time of urination is recorded.
4. Immediately after this voiding, venous blood is withdrawn and 5 cc. placed in an oxalate bottle.
5. Two and one-half hours after starting the test, the patient again empties the bladder completely into a clean, dry bottle. The exact time of urination is recorded.
6. If the patient is unable to urinate at the specified times, the test may still be performed, provided exact times of urination are recorded.

Laboratory Procedure. The urea concentration of the blood and urine samples are measured as described under *Urea Nitrogen, Chapter 3*. From these measurements, the volume of blood cleared of urea by one minute's urinary excretion is calculated and expressed as a percentage of standard clearance.

Normal Range. 75 to 130 per cent.

Urobilinogen

This is a test to aid in the differential diagnosis between complete and incomplete obstruction of the biliary tract. Increases in urinary urobilinogen (a breakdown product of hemoglobin) occur in many conditions, including hemolytic diseases, liver damage and severe infections. However, in complete obstructive jaundice without infection there is ordinarily no excess of urobilinogen in the urine.

Procedure for Collecting Specimen. A urine sample is placed in a bottle and sent to the laboratory. In some institutions a random sample of urine may be used; in others a 2-hour morning specimen or a 24-hour urine may be tested.

Laboratory Procedure. To serial dilutions of the urine sample is added Ehrlich's reagent. The greatest dilution giving a pink color is determined.

Normal Range. A positive reaction at 1:20 dilution of the urine.

6

Tests Performed on Feces

Although relatively few tests are done on feces, those which are performed are important to the patient whose health or life may depend on an accurate diagnosis based on such an examination. Careful collection and handling of the specimen and expert, conscientious performance of the examination are as essential as in any other test.

Blood

The discovery of blood in the feces may uncover a serious bleeding lesion of the gastrointestinal tract. Blood from a lesion in the lower colon is bright red and readily recognized. However, blood coming from the stomach or small intestine is so changed by the digestive process that it is not recognizable on inspection. Therefore, chemical tests are performed to see if there is occult blood in the feces.

Procedure for Collecting Specimen. Sometimes, any random stool is used. At other times, since meat may also give a positive result, the physician may order the test after the patient has been on a meat-free diet for 3 days.

Laboratory Procedure. To the stool is added either

benzidine or guaiac. A blue color represents a positive result.

Normal Range. On a regular diet, many persons normally have positive benzidine or guaiac tests. Even on a meat-free diet, some people will normally show a positive test from gums which bleed when brushing the teeth.

Parasites

Examinations of feces for parasites are performed in order to identify the parasites or their eggs. The therapy will usually depend on the type of parasite found, so that precise identification is important.

Procedure for Collecting Specimen. The sample of feces is obtained and kept in various ways, depending on the type of parasite sought. Oily cathartics are never given. An ordinary "cold" stool is suitable for examination for ova and for amebic and similar cysts. A "warm" stool, which is kept at approximately body temperature until delivery at the laboratory, is suitable for all the previous examinations and also for trophozoites (mobile forms). A proctoscopic aspiration or scraping may be tested for trophozoites. A proctoscopic biopsy may be done for Schistosome ova. Anal swabs are done for pinworm eggs. All samples are brought to the laboratory at once.

Laboratory Procedure. The stool samples are examined microscopically and parasites and ova identified.

Normal Range. A large percentage of the population harbors harmless parasites like E. coli and certain flagellates.

Undigested Food

The finding of large amounts of undigested food may indicate some abnormality of digestion.

Procedure for Collecting Specimen. A stool specimen is placed in a container which is covered tightly.

Laboratory Procedure. The specimen is examined macroscopically and, if requested, chemical tests for starch and fat may be performed.

Normal Range. There is usually a small residue of undigested food in all feces.

Urobilin

Normally there are considerable amounts of urobilin (also called stercobilin) in the feces. However, in complete obstruction of the bile passages, the feces contain no urobilin and are lighter than usual, often clay colored. This test may be useful in diagnosing complete biliary obstruction and in ascertaining when the obstruction becomes partially relieved.

Procedure for Collecting Specimen. A stool specimen is placed in a container which is covered tightly.

Laboratory Procedure. A sample of the feces is mixed with a saturated solution of mercuric chloride. Urobilin will produce a deep red color after an interval of 6 to 24 hours.

Normal Range. There is usually considerable urobilin in the feces.

7

Miscellaneous Tests

The following tests do not fall into any of the preceding categories. They measure important aspects of body function and are likely to be ordered frequently.

Basal Metabolic Rate (B.M.R.)

This test gives an indication of the rate at which metabolic processes take place under standard conditions. The basal metabolic rate may be elevated in such conditions as hyperthyroidism, anxiety and infection. It may be lowered in hypothyroidism and during sedation.

Although the B.M.R. is being replaced by other tests, it remains useful in many situations when properly performed.

Procedure for Performing Test. The patient, from the outset, must understand the test procedure thoroughly since any anxiety about it might change the basal metabolic rate. He should have a good night's sleep before the test and must fast from 10 p.m. until after the test. He may take water. In the test the patient lies on a comfortable cot and breathes pure oxygen. The B.M.R. machine records the amount of oxygen used per unit of time. From this the basal metabolic rate is calculated.

Normal Range.–20% to +20%.

Biopsy

Biopsies are examinations of tissue specimen removed from the patient. They may be performed on many kinds of tissue from almost any area. Biopsies may be done to help diagnose various conditions, including malignancies.

Procedure for Collecting Specimen. The doctor removes the specimen, using whatever technique is appropriate. A biopsy is a surgical procedure requiring strictest precautions.

Laboratory Procedure. The tissue specimen is fixed, sectioned, stained and examined microscopically by a pathologist. In some cases, in order to save time, examination of a frozen section may be performed.

Capillary Fragility

See Tourniquet Test for Capillary Fragility

Chloride in Sweat

This is a test for cystic fibrosis of the pancreas. It has been found that children with cystic fibrosis excrete much greater amounts of chloride in their perspiration than do normal children. Therefore, if an excessively high concentration of chloride is found in the sweat, the presumptive diagnosis becomes cystic fibrosis, and the child is treated accordingly.

Some institutions use this test in a simplified form as a routine screening test in all children. It is hoped that the test will uncover early cases which can then be treated more effectively.

Procedure for Performing Test. The child's hands are washed and dried. They are then kept from contact with other parts of the body for 15 minutes. After that interval a test paper, impregnated with silver chromate, is moistened with distilled or tap water (*not* saline), and the patient's hand is pressed down on the paper for 4 seconds. The print is then compared to that of a normal child. Wherever chloride is present, the red silver chromate changes to white silver chloride. The imprint of the normal child's hand is indistinct, while the imprint of the hand of the child with cystic fibrosis is heavy and distinct.

Normal Range. Hand print is light and indistinct.

Electrocardiogram (E.C.G.)

The electrocardiogram records the electrical potentials produced by the heart. All cells possess bioelectricity. Very sensitive instruments can pick up a difference of potential between the inside and outside of any living cell. With muscle and nerve cells, following stimulation, the cell membrane becomes permeable to certain ions, and a current flows between the inside and outside of the cell. The difference in potential travels as a wave down the cell. Our knowledge of the exact mechanisms involved is still incomplete, although most scientists believe they consist of depolarization and repolarization of the cell membrane. The electrocardiograph is a sensitive instrument, recording the changes in electrical potential of the heart which are transmitted through the limbs and chest wall. The record itself is called the *electrocardiogram*. It should be noted that only electrical potentials are measured. These electrical potentials are not directly related to force of contraction. Therefore, the electrocardiogram gives no indication as to the strength of the heart. In fact, it is possible, experimentally, to record a normal looking electrocardiogram from a heart so weakened that no contraction whatever can be observed or recorded. The electrocardiogram is useful in diagnosing cardiac arrhythmias and in diagnosing and following the course of myocardial infarctions. Electrocardiograms are interpreted by physicians with special training.

Procedure for Performing Test. Appropriate electrodes are strapped to the patient's limbs and chest and connected to the machine which records the tracing. There are many varieties of electrocardiographs and each is operated somewhat differently from the others.

Normal Range. The cardiologist decides whether the tracing is normal.

Electroencephalogram (E.E.G.)

This is a record of the electrical potentials produced by the brain cells. It may be used in the diagnosis of epilepsy and similar disorders. It is far more complex than the electrocardiogram. The electrical potentials which are recorded from the brain may be 100 times weaker than those recorded by the electrocardiogram, so that a much more sensitive instrument (electroencephalograph) is required to record them. Special precautions must be taken against electrical interference.

Procedure for Performing Test. Electrodes are fastened to the patient's scalp and connected to the machine which records the tracing.

Normal Range. The neurologist decides whether the tracing is normal.

Gastric Analysis (Tube)

This test is performed to determine the degree of acidity of stomach contents. It is an uncomfortable procedure for most patients, so that newer tests of gastric acidity, using various resins, have been devised. Nevertheless, gastric analysis is still utilized in many institutions.

The stomach ordinarily secretes hydrochloric acid to aid in digestion. In certain conditions, such as duodenal or gastric ulcer, the quantity of acid may be greater than normal. In other conditions, such as pernicious anemia, gastric carcinoma and simple achlorhydria, there may be none of the acid. Occasionally, the gastric contents may be examined for enzymes, tissue fragments and tubercle bacilli.

Procedure for Collecting Specimen. The patient receives nothing by mouth after supper on the night before the test, unless ordered by the doctor. The physician coats a cold Levin tube with mineral oil, inserts it into the patient's mouth or nose, and passes it down the esophagus into the stomach. An emesis basin is always kept at hand since some patients become nauseated. After insertion of the Levin tube the physician sucks out the stomach contents with a large syringe, and subsequently stimulates gastric secretion. The latter may be accomplished by feeding the patient a test meal or by injecting insulin or histamine. Samples of the gastric contents are then removed every 15 minutes for 1 hour.

Laboratory Procedure. The samples of gastric juice are first tested for free hydrochloric acid and then for total hydrochloric acid content, including that bound to other substances. In each case the gastric juice sample is titrated with sodium hydroxide in the presence of reagents which change color at specific pHs.

Normal Range. Usually 100 to 170 degrees of acidity, but 8 per cent of healthy persons have no acid. The normal range depends on the type of stimulus used to induce gastric secretion. The total acidity is usually up to 20 degrees greater than the free acidity. A degree of acidity represents the number of cc. of 1/10 normal sodium hydroxide needed to neutralize 100 cc. of gastric juice. It is also equivalent to 3.65 mg. of hydrochloric acid.

Gastric Analysis (Tubeless)

This method of determining the presence of stomach acid does not require the passing of a tube into the esophagus and is more comfortable for the patient. It is based on the fact that free hydrochloric acid will displace certain materials from combination with other substances. The earlier tubeless analyses were performed with quininium resin indicator. More recently, an azure indicator dye has been used.

In general this method is not suitable for exact quantitative analysis but gives the essential information needed in many cases, i.e., whether free acid is present in the stomach. Since false negative reactions sometimes occur, a negative report is not diagnostic of achlorhydria unless confirmed by standard gastric analysis. The tubeless method is useful because it can save most patients from the discomfort of intubation.

Quininium Resin Indicator

Procedure for Collecting Specimen. No drugs or vitamins are administered for at least 24 hours before the test. Quinine and quinidine should not be given for 3 days before the test. No food is taken after midnight. In the morning the patient urinates and the specimen is discarded. He is then given 250 mg. of caffeine sodium benzoate to stimulate gastric secretion. After 1 hour he urinates and the specimen is saved. He then swallows the contents of 1 packet of quininium resin with one-half glass of water. At the end of 2 hours a urine specimen is collected and sent to the laboratory.

Laboratory Procedure. The urine sample is alkalinized and an ether extract made. The extract is acidified with sulfuric acid and the solution placed under ultraviolet light. Flurorescence indicates quinine. The amount of quinine is estimated roughly by comparison with standards.

Normal Range. More than 25 microgm. of quinine in the urine sample indicates free hydrochloric acid in the stomach.

Azure Indicator Dye

Procedure for Collecting Specimen. No food is taken after midnight but water is permitted. In the morning, the first urine specimen is discarded. The patient is then given a glass of water with 500 mg. of caffeine sodium benzoate. After one hour he urinates, and the urine specimen is saved as a control. He then swallows the blue granules of the dye in one-half glass of water. After an additional 2 hours he urinates, and the urine is sent to the laboratory. The urine may be blue or green for several days after. This has no significance.

Laboratory Procedure. Both urine specimens are diluted to 300 cc., and 10 cc. aliquots are compared to standards.

Normal Range. A blue color equal to or more than 0.6 mg. standard indicates the presence of free hydrochloric acid in the stomach.

Microscopic Tests for Malignant Cells (Papanicolaou Smear)

In many areas of the body malignant (cancer) cells separate from tumors and may be identified microscopically. This may make possible the diagnosis of malignancy early enough for satisfactory treatment or even complete cure. Such tests are most commonly performed on the female genital tract but are also of value in other areas. Other specimens include bronchial, esophageal, rectal, and colonic washings, duodenal drainage, gastric and nipple secretions, pleural, peritoneal and pericardial exudates, prostate smears, sputum and urine.

Procedure for Collecting Specimen. The physician collects the specimen. If it consists of a washing, drainage, exudate, aspiration fluid or urine, it is mixed with equal parts of 95% alcohol and sent to the laboratory. If it consists of a smear or a secretion, it is smeared on a glass slide which is then immersed in a solution containing equal parts of 95% alcohol and ether *before the smear can dry*. Sputum is collected in 70% alcohol.

Laboratory Procedure. The fluid specimens are concentrated by centrifugation and smeared. All smears are stained and examined microscopically.

Normal Range. No malignant cells are found normally.

Papanicolaou Smear —*See above*

Sputum Smears for Eosinophiles and Elastic Fibers

The sputum contains eosinophiles in cases of allergic asthma, but not in "cardiac" asthma. Finding eosinophiles may, therefore, aid in the differential diagnosis between these two conditions. If elastic fibers are found in the smear, there is probably a destructive lesion of the walls of the alveoli or bronchioles, such as tuberculosis with cavitation, malignancy, or lung abscess.

Procedure for Collecting Specimen. Sputum is collected in a container which is then covered. In some institutions the sputum is smeared on 2 slides in the patient's room. Elsewhere, the smearing is done in the laboratory.

Laboratory Procedure. The slides are stained and examined microscopically for eosinophiles and elastic fibers.

Normal Range. Normally there are very few, if any, eosinophiles or elastic fibers in the sputum.

Tourniquet Test for Capillary Fragility

This test measures the ability of the capillaries to remain intact under stress. Increased capillary fragility may be found in many types of systemic vascular abnormalities, including scurvy, thrombocytopenic purpura, and purpura accompanying severe infections.

Procedure for Performing Test. The physician inflates a blood pressure cuff on the patient's arm to a point midway between diastolic and systolic pressures. The pressure is maintained for 10 minutes. Any petechiae (small hemorrhages under the skin) render the test positive. Sometimes counts of petechiae per unit of area may also be reported.

Normal Range. Some people will normally have a positive test, particularly those with red hair.

Xylose —*See Oral d-xylose Tolerance Test*

8

Normal Values in Infants and Children

In infants and children the normal values for many laboratory tests differ considerably from those of adults. In the body of this book the values given are for adults. In this section, however, the important differences in the values for infants and children will be considered.

Blood

At birth, the infant usually has a higher hemoglobin content than the adult. The average is about 17 Gm. per 100 cc., but higher concentrations are normal. This high level falls rapidly. At the age of 2 months it is about 14 Gm. per 100 cc., and at about 3 months it reaches a low point of about 11 Gm. per 100 cc. Thereafter, the hemoglobin content tends to rise very slowly, reaching about 13 Gm. per 100 cc. at the age of 2 years.

The red blood cells follow a similar pattern.

The white blood cells (leucocytes) are very numerous at birth. They average 20,000 per $mm.^3$ of blood, but counts as high as 35,000 per $mm.^3$ are normal. This is about 4 times the adult level. The leucocyte count falls gradually but remains higher than the adult level for at least the first 2 years of life. Accordingly, an elevated leucocyte count in a young infant has little or no diagnostic significance.

The infant normally has some degree of icterus with an elevated serum bilirubin from the second day to the seventh. This results from two factors—a considerable degree of destruction of the red blood cells and immaturity of the liver.

On the other hand, an excessive degree of icterus or visible icterus within 24 hours of birth may denote a serious condition, such as erythroblastosis fetalis (Chapter 3: Blood Types/Rh factor) which requires prompt, efficient therapy.

In newborn infants a low fasting blood glucose, about 50 mgm. per 100 cc., or sometimes even lower, is common. This rises gradually, reaching 75 mgm. per 100 cc. in the small child.

The total cholesterol in newborn infants is quite low, ranging from 80 to 165 mgm. per 100 cc. of blood. However, this level rises until, in most children, it reaches 200 to 300 mgm. per 100 cc. This is higher than usual adult levels. It may not be a strictly physiologic change. There is a strong likelihood that the high serum cholesterol levels in American children result from their high intake of dairy products after the age of weaning.

The alkaline phosphatase levels are high, up to 20 Bodansky units because of the formation of new bone cells.

During the first few days of life the level of blood urea nitrogen may be as high 40 mgm. per 100 cc., of blood. However, it rapidly falls to the adult level.

In the newborn the blood potassium level may be as high as 7 milliequivalents per liter. It, too, soon drops to adult levels.

Urine

Albuminuria is a common, almost universal, finding in infants during the first week or two of life. In older children it may or may not indicate the presence of disease.

Infants and children under 8 years of age normally excrete practically no 17-ketosteroids. At the age of 8, excretion increases gradually, reaching adult levels at about age 18. Increased levels in infants and young children may result from adrenal hyperplasia.

Cerebrospinal Fluid

In the newborn the glucose levels in the cerebrospinal fluid may normally be as low as 35 mgm. per 100 cc. This, of course, is correlated with the low blood glucose levels. As the blood glucose levels rise, so do the C.S.F. levels.

PART TWO: TABLES

9

Tests Listed by Organs or Systems

Table 1

Tests of Blood Function and Blood Disorders

Test	*Performed on*
A/G ratio	Blood serum
Albumin	Blood serum
Bilirubin, partition	Blood serum
Bilirubin, total	Blood serum
Bleeding time	Capillaries of skin
Blood counts	Whole blood
Blood culture	Whole blood
Blood types	Whole blood
Calcium	Blood serum
Clotting time	Whole blood
CO_2 combining power	Blood serum
Fibrinogen	Blood plasma
Globulin	Blood serum
Hematocrit	Whole blood
Hemoglobin	Whole blood
Icterus index	Blood serum
Malaria film	Whole blood
Methemoglobin	Whole blood
pH	Blood serum
Platelet count	Whole blood
Porphyrins	Urine
Potassium	Blood serum
Protein	Blood serum
Prothrombin time	Blood serum
Red cell fragility	Whole blood
Reticulocyte count	Whole blood
Sedimentation rate	Whole blood
Sickle cell test	Whole blood
Sodium	Blood serum
Sulfhemoglobin	Whole blood
Tourniquet test for capillary fragility	Capillaries of skin of arm
Urinary blood	Urine

Table 2

Tests of Liver Function and Liver Disorders

Test	*Performed on*
A/G ratio	Blood serum
Bilirubin, partition	Blood serum
Bilirubin, total	Blood serum
Bromsulphalein retention (B.S.P.)	Blood serum
Cephalin flocculation	Blood serum
Cholesterol	Blood serum
Cholesterol esters	Blood serum
Fecal urobilin	Feces
Glucose	Blood serum
Glucose tolerance	Blood serum and urine
Icterus index	Blood serum
Phosphatase, alkaline	Blood serum
Prothrombin time	Blood serum
Serum transaminase	Blood serum
Thymol turbidity	Blood serum
Urinary bile and bilirubin	Urine
Urobilinogen	Urine

Table 3

Tests of Kidney Function and Kidney Disorders

Test	*Performed on*
Addis	Urine
Albumin, globulin, A/G ratio and protein	Blood serum
Albumin (qualitative and quantitative) in urine	Urine
Calcium	Blood serum
Chlorides	Blood serum
CO_2 combining power	Blood serum
Concentration and dilution	Urine
Creatinine	Blood serum
Microscopic tests of urinary sediment	Urine
Non-protein nitrogen (N.P.N.)	Blood serum
Phenolsulfonphthalein (P.S.P.)	Urine
Phosphorus	Blood serum
Potassium	Blood serum
Sodium	Blood serum
Specific gravity	Urine
Urea clearance	Blood serum and urine
Urea nitrogen	Blood serum

Table 4

Tests of Metabolic Function and Metabolic Disorders

Test	*Performed on*
Acetone	Urine
Ascorbic acid	Blood plasma
Ascorbic acid tolerance	Urine
Basal metabolic rate (B.M.R.)	Patient
Calcium	Blood serum
Diacetic (aceto-acetic) acid	Urine
Fermentation test for sugar	Urine
Glucose	Blood serum
Glucose tolerance	Blood serum and urine
pH	Blood serum
Phenylketonuria	Urine
Sugar, qualitative and quantitative	Urine
Uric acid	Blood serum

Table 5

Tests for Infections, Microorganisms, and Resistance to Microorganisms

Test	*Performed on*
Agglutination	Blood serum
Anti-streptolysin O titer	Blood serum
Blood culture	Whole blood
C-reactive protein	Blood serum
Colloidal gold	Spinal fluid
Heterophile antibody	Blood serum
Malaria film	Whole blood
Miscellaneous fluid cultures	Body fluids
Nose and throat culture	Nose and throat secretions
Parasites	Stool
Sedimentation rate	Whole blood
Serological tests	Blood serum and spinal fluid
Special tests	Spinal fluid
Spinal fluid chlorides	Spinal fluid
Spinal fluid culture	Spinal fluid
Spinal fluid protein	Spinal fluid
Spinal fluid sugar	Spinal fluid
Sputum culture and smear	Sputum
Stool culture	Stool
Urine culture	Urine
White cell differential count	Whole blood
Wound culture	Wound exudates

Table 6

Tests for Malignancy

Test	*Type of Malignancy*	*Performed on*
Aschheim-Zondek, quantitative	Teratoma	Urine
Bence-Jones protein	Bone tumors	Urine
Melanin	Melanomas	Urine
Microscopic tests	All	Various fluids
Papanicolaou (see Microscopic tests)		
Phosphatase, acid	Prostate carcinoma	Blood serum
Phosphatase, alkaline	Bone tumors	Blood serum

Table 7

Tests of Endocrine Glands and Their Function

Test	*Gland*	*Performed on*
Amylase	Pancreas	Blood serum
Calcium	Parathyroid	Blood serum
Calcium (Sulkowitch)	Parathyroid	Urine
Cholesterol, total	Thyroid	Blood serum
Glucose (Sugar)	Pancreas	Blood serum and urine
Glucose tolerance	Pancreas	Blood serum and urine
Insulin tolerance	Pituitary and thyroid	Blood serum
17-ketosteroid excretion	Adrenal cortex	Urine
Lipase	Pancreas	Blood serum
Phosphorus	Parathyroid	Blood serum
Potassium	Adrenal cortex	Blood serum
Protein-bound iodine (P.B.I.)	Thyroid	Blood serum
Sodium	Adrenal cortex	Blood serum

Table 8

Tests for Poisoning

Test	*Performed on*
Carbon monoxide	Whole blood
Lead	Urine
Methemoglobin	Whole blood
Porphyrins	Urine
Sulfhemoglobin	Whole blood

Table 9

Miscellaneous Tests

Test	*Performed on*
Aschheim-Zondek	Urine
Chloride in sweat	Sweat
Congo red retention	Blood serum
Electrocardiogram (E.C.G.)	Patient
Electroencephalogram (E.E.G.)	Patient
Fecal blood	Feces
Friedman (pregnancy)	Urine
Gastric analysis	Gastric juice
Lupus erythematosus cell test (L.E.)	Whole blood
Oral d-xylose tolerance	Urine
Sulfonamide level	Blood serum
Urinary chlorides	Urine

10

Quick Reference Tables

Table 1

Tests Performed on Venous Blood

Test	*Cc. of blood*	*Container*	*Anticoagulant*	*Normal Range (Adults)*
A/G ratio (see Albumin)				
Agglutination	5	Test tube	None	See test
Albumin, globulin, protein, A/G ratio	6 (total)	Test tube	None	3.2 to 5.6 Gm./100 cc. 1.3 to 3.2 Gm./100 cc. 6.0 to 8.0 Gm./100 cc. 1.5:1 to 2.5:1
Amylase	6	Test tube	None	80 to 150 units (Somogyi)
Anti-streptolysin O titer	5	Test tube	None	Up to 200 units/cc. of serum
Ascorbic acid	6	Oxalate bottle	Oxalate	0.7 to 1.4 Gm./100 cc. of plasma
Bilirubin	5	Test tube	None	0.1 to 1.0 mg./100 cc. of serum
Blood types	5	Test tube	None	—
Blood urea nitrogen (B.U.N.) (see Urea nitrogen)				
Bromsulphalein (B.S.P.)	5	Test tube	None	Less than 0.4 mg./100 cc. of serum
Calcium	6	Test tube	None	9.0 to 11.5 mg./100 cc. of serum
Carbon monoxide	5	Oxalate bottle	Oxalate	Less than 0.8 vol. %
Cephalin flocculation	5	Test tube	None	0 to 1+

Test	*Cc. of blood*	*Container*	*Anticoagulant*	*Normal Range (Adults)*
Chlorides	5	Test tube	None	100 to 106 mEq./l. of serum, or 355 to 376 mg. chloride /100 cc. of serum
Cholesterol	5	Test tube	None	120 to 260 mg./100 cc. of serum
Cholesterol esters	7	Test tube	None	68% to 78% of total cholesterol
Clotting time	4	4 small test tubes	None	According to method
CO_2 combining power	8	Test tube with oil	None	56 to 70 vol./100 of serum or 25 to 31 millimols/liter of serum
Congo red retention	6	Test tube	None	Less than 40% disappears from blood in 1 hr.
C-reactive protein	5	Test tube	None	None
Creatinine	6	Test tube	None	0.6 to 1.3 mg./100 cc.
Fibrinogen	5	Oxalate bottle	Oxalate	200 to 600 mg./100 cc. plasma
Globulin (see Albumin)				
Glucose	3-5	Oxalate bottle	Oxalate	70 to 105 mg./100 cc. of serum
Glucose tolerance (oral)	3 per sample	Oxalate bottle	Oxalate	Peak under 150 mg./100 cc. of serum
Glucose tolerance (intravenous)	3 per sample	Oxalate bottle	Oxalate	Return to fasting level within 1 hr.
Hematocrit	4	Oxalate bottle	Oxalate	Women, 35% to 45%; men 40% to 50% of blood volume

Table 1 (*continued*)

Tests Performed on Venous Blood

Test	*Cc. of blood*	*Container*	*Anticoagulant*	*Normal Range (Adults)*
Heterophile antibody	5	Test tube	None	Concentrations up to 1/28.
Icterus index	5	Test tube	None	4 to 6 units
Insulin tolerance	3 per sample	Fluoride bottle	Fluoride	Return to pre-injection level within 2 hrs.
Lipase	6	Test tube	None	1.5 units or less
Lupus erythematosus cell test (L.E.)	5	Oxalate bottle	Oxalate	None
Methemoglobin	5	Oxalate bottle	Oxalate	None
Non-protein nitrogen (N.P.N.)	5	Oxalate bottle	Oxalate	15 to 35 mg./100 cc. of serum
pH	5	Test tube with oil	None	7.35 to 7.45
Phosphatase, acid	5	2 test tubes	None	Less than 2.5 King-Armstrong units, or less than 1.5 phenol units
Phosphatase, alkaline	5	2 test tubes	None	Adults 1.5-4, children less than 20 Bodansky units
Phosphorus	4	Test tube	None	Adults 3.0-4.5 mg./100 cc. of serum, children 4 to 6.5 mg./100 cc. of serum
Potassium*	6	Test tube with oil	None	4 to 5 mEq./l.

Test	*Cc. of blood*	*Container*	*Anticoagulant*	*Normal Range (Adults)*
Protein (see Albumin)				
Protein-bound iodine (P.B.I.)	8	Test tube	None	3.0 to 8.0 mcgm/100 cc. of serum
Prothrombin time	4.5	Special test tube	Special oxalate solution	11 to 18 seconds = 100%
Red cell fragility	5	Oxalate bottle	Oxalate	Complete hemolysis between 30% and 0.36% NaCl (see test)
Sedimentation rate	4	Oxalate bottle	Oxalate	Men 0 to 15 mm./hr., women 0 to 20 mm./hr. (see test)
Serology	5	Test tube	None	See test
Serology	5	Test tube	None	See test
Serum transaminase	5	Test tube	None	Up to 40 units
Sodium*	6	Test tube with oil	None	138 to 145 mEq./l of serum
Sugar (see Glucose)				
Sulfhemoglobin	5	Oxalate bottle	Oxalate	None
Sulfonamide	5	Oxalate bottle	Oxalate	None
Thymol turbidity	5	Test tube	None	Less than 5 units
Urea nitrogen	5	Oxalate bottle	Oxalate	9 to 17 mg./100 cc. of blood
Uric acid	5	Oxalate bottle	Oxalate	3.5 to 6.0 mg./100 cc. of serum

*Use oiled syringe

Table 2

Tests Performed on Capillary Blood

(From Finger or Ear Lobe)

Test	*Normal Range*
Bleeding time	1 to 6 minutes
Hemoglobin	12 to 18 Gm./100 cc. of blood
Platelet count	200,000 to 500,000/cubic mm. of blood
Red cell count	4 to 6 million/cubic mm. of blood
Reticulocyte count	0.1 to 4.0/100 red blood cells
White cell count	4,000 to 11,000/cubic mm. of blood
White cell differential count	Neutrophiles 54% to 62% Eosinophiles 1% to 3% Basophiles 0% to 1% Lymphocytes 25% to 33% Monocytes 0% to 9%

Table 3

Tests Performed on Cerebrospinal Fluid

Test	*Cc. of Fluid*	*Normal Range*
Chlorides	2	720 to 760 mg. NaCl/100 cc.
Colloidal gold	1	All 0 or few 1+ precipitations
Culture	2	Negative
Protein	2	15 to 40 mg./100 cc.
Serology	7	Negative
Sugar	2	50 to 80 mg./100 cc.

Table 4

Tests Performed on Urine

Test	*Urine Sample*	*Normal Range*
Aceto-acetic acid (see Diacetic Acid)		
Acetone	Random	None
Addis test	12-hr. specimen	Red cells 0 to 450,000 White cells 30,000 to 1,000,000 Hyaline casts 0 to 5,000 } per 12-hr. specimen
Albumin, qualitative*	Random	None or small amounts
Aschheim-Zondek	Morning specimen	Negative
Ascorbic acid tolerance	24-hr. specimen	About 30% of amount administered
Bence-Jones protein	Random	None
Bile and bilirubin	Random	None
Blood	Random	None (see test)
Calcium (Sulkowitch)	Random	A fine white precipitate
Chlorides, quantitative	24-hr. specimen	See test
Concentration and dilution	Several, at specified intervals (see test)	Concentration: specific gravity 1.026 or higher; Dilution: specific gravity 1,003
Diacetic (aceto-acetic) acid	Random	None

Test	*Urine Sample*	*Normal Range*
Fermentation test for sugar	Random	None
Friedman (pregnancy)	Morning specimen	Negative
17-ketosteroid excretion	24-hr. specimen	Males, 8 to 20 mg./24 hrs., Females, 5 to 15 mg./24 hrs.
Lead	24-hr. specimen	.020 to .080 mg./liter
Melanin	Random	None
Microscopic*	Random	See test
Oral d-xylose tolerance	5-hr. total, minimum 150 cc.	5 to 8 Gm. within 5 hrs. after ingestion
pH*	Random	4.8 to 8.0
Phenolsulfonphthalein (P.S.P.)	Several, at specified intervals (see test)	Elimination of 63% to 84% in 2 hrs.
Phenylketonuria	Random	None
Porphyrins	24-hr. specimen	Minute amounts
Specific gravity*	Random	1.001 to 1.030
Sugar, qualitative*	Random	None
Sugar, quantitative	24-hr. specimen	None
Urea clearance	Several, at specified intervals (see test)	75% to 130%
Urobilinogen	Differs in different institutions (see test)	Positive reaction at 1:20 dilution

* Part of routine urinalysis

Table 5

Tests Performed on Feces

Test	*Fecal Specimen*	*Normal Range*
Blood (guiac or benzidine)	Random, or following meat-free diet, as ordered	May be positive on random specimen
Parasites	As ordered (see test)	Harmless parasites such as E. coli and flagellates are normal
Undigested food	Random	Small amounts
Urobilin	Random	Large amounts

Table 6

Miscellaneous Tests

Test	*Specimen*	*Normal Range*
Basal metabolic rate (B.M.R.)	Patient	–20% to +20%
Chloride in sweat	Hand (see test)	Light, indistinct hand print
Gastric analysis	Gastric fluid	Depends on stimulus (see test)
Gastric analysis, tubeless	2-hr. urine specimen (see test)	More than 25 microgm. quinine or blue color not less than 0.6 mgm. azure A standard
Electrocardiogram (E.C.G.)	Patient	Interpretation by cardiologist
Electroencephalogram (E.E.G.)	Patient	Interpretation by neurologist
Microscopic tests for malignant cells	Various body fluids	None
Sputum smears	Sputum	Few eosinophiles or elastic fibers
Tourniquet for capillary fragility	Capillaries of skin of arm	Usually negative

Table 7

Iodine-Containing Drugs and Diagnostic Agents (Partial List)

Material	*Manufacturer*
Amend's solution	Leeming
Arocalcin tablets	Pitman-Moore
Bronchoid Jr.	Moore
Calathesin	Walker
Calcidrine	Abbott
Ceradine	Ulmer
Cher-Iomine	Pitman-Moore
Child's Drikof	Walker
Cholografin	Squibb
Creodide	Maltbie; Wallace & Tiernan
Di-iodo Tyrosine	Organon
Diodrast	Winthrop
Endoarsan	Endo
Entero-Vioform	Ciba
Entodon	Winthrop
Felsol powders and tablets	American Felsol
Floraquin	Searle
Iocapral	Winthrop
Iocylate tablets	Pitman-Moore
Iod-Ethamine tablets	Pitman-Moore
Iodex	Menley & James

Table 7 (*continued*)

Material	*Manufacturer*
Iodized Petrogen	Wyeth
Iodochlorol	Searle
Iodo-Ichthyol	Ulmer
Iosalex ointment	Pitman-Moore
Itrumil	Ciba
Limodin	Central
Lipoiodine	Ciba
Milpath	Wallace
Miokon sodium	Mallinckrodt
Nail polish	Several manufacturers
Organidin	Wampole
Oridine	Lilly
Quadrinal	Knoll
Quin-O-Creme	Walker
Skiodan	Winthrop
Sodium iodide	Several manufacturers
Tamponets	Walker
Telepaque	Winthrop
Thixokon	Mallinckrodt
Thyractin	Winthrop
Tincture of iodine	Several manufacturers
Urokon sodium	Mallinckrodt
Vioform	Ciba
Vitamin combinations	Many manufacturers

Table 8

Laboratory Aids and Materials for Rapid, Simplified Laboratory Tests

These aids will be helpful in rapid office and bedside diagnostic procedures; some of them are also useful in hospital emergency rooms. Most tests give rough quantitative measurements. Inclusion in this list does not constitute an endorsement. For details about each test write to the manufacturer.

Tests of Blood	*Material*	*Type*	*Manufacturer*
Culture	Blood culture outfit	Composite	Lederle
Acetoacetic acid	Ketostix	Paper strip	Ames
Ketone bodies	Acetest	Tablet	Ames
Phosphatase, acid	Phosphatabs, acid	Tablet	Warner-Chilcott
Phosphatase, alkaline	Phosphatabs, alkaline	Tablet	Warner-Chilcott
Glucose	Dextrotest	Tablet	Ames
Glucose	Blood sugar screening test	Test kit	Lilly

Tests of Urine	*Material*	*Type*	*Manufacturer*
Acetoacetic acid	Ketostix	Paper strip	Ames
Albumin	Albustix	Paper strip	Ames
"	Albutest	Tablet	Ames
"	Bumintest	Tablet	Ames
"	Bromalin	Solution	Crookes-Barnes
"	Albumin test solution	Solution	Endo

Table 8 (*continued*)

Bilirubin	Ictotest	Tablet	Ames
Blood & hemoglobin	Occultest	Tablet	Ames
Glucose	Tes-Tape	Paper strip	Lilly
Glucose	Clinistix	Paper strip	Ames
"	Clinitest	Tablet	Ames
Glucose & protein	Uristix	Paper strip	Ames
Ketone bodies	Acetest	Tablet	Ames
pH	Nitrazine paper	Paper strip	Squibb
Phenylketones	Phenistix	Paper strip	Ames

Tests of Feces	*Material*	*Type*	*Manufacturer*
Blood	Hematest	Tablet	Ames

Tests of Bacterial Sensitivity	*Material*	*Type*	*Manufacturer*
Sensitivity disc	Sensitivity disc	Paper overlay	Difco
" "	Unidisc	Paper overlay	Difco

Miscellaneous Aids	*Material*	*Type*	*Manufacturer*
Anticoagulant tablet	EDTAP	Tablet	Standard Scientific Supply

SUPPLEMENT

units of measurement

needles, syringes, venipuncture

11

Units of Measurement Used in Clinical Laboratory Procedures

A *gram* (Gm.) is a standard unit of weight or mass. It is equivalent to 1/28 ounce.

A *milligram* (mg., mgm.) is 1/1000 of a gram.

A *microgram* (microgm., mcgm., gamma) is 1/1,000,000 of a gram.

A *milligram per cent* is a milligram per 100 cubic centimeters or per 100 grams.

A *cubic centimeter* (cc.) is a unit of volume equal to a cube 1 centimeter in each dimension. It is equivalent to a milliliter (1/1000 of a liter).

A *cubic millimeter* (mm^3) is a unit of volume equal to a cube 1 millimeter in each dimension. It is equivalent to 1/1000 of a cubic centimeter.

A *liter* (l.) is a unit of liquid measurement. It is equivalent to 1000 cubic centimeters, or about 1 quart.

A *volume per cent* is a measurement of the amount of gas dissolved in a liquid. For example, when 10 cc. of gas is dissolved in 100 cc. of fluid, the concentration can be expressed as 10 volumes per cent.

A *mol* is the number of grams equal to the number expressing the molecular weight of the substance. Since sodium, for example, has a weight of 23, a mol of sodium is 23 grams.

A *molar* solution is a mol of a substance dissolved in enough fluid to make 1 liter of solution. Thus a molar solution of sodium has 23 grams of sodium ion per liter.

A *millimol* is 1/1000 of a mol. A millimol of sodium is 23 milligrams.

A *millimolar* solution is a millimol of a substance dissolved in enough fluid to make 1 liter of solution. A millimolar solution of sodium contains 23 milligrams of sodium ion per liter.

An *equivalent* is a mol divided by a valence. An equivalent of sodium is 23/1 or 23 grams. An equivalent of calcium (weight 40, valence 2) is 40/2 or 20 grams.

A *milliequivalent* (mEq.) is 1/1000 of an equivalent. A milliequivalent of sodium is 23 milligrams and a milliequivalent of calcium is 20 milligrams.

A *degree of acidity* is the amount of acid contained in 100 cc. of gastric juice which will just neutralize 1 cc. of 1/10 normal sodium hydroxide solution. A degree of acidity is equivalent to 3.65 mg. of hydrochloric acid. This unit of measurement is used in describing the acidity of gastric juice.

A *unit* is an arbitrary measurement used when no other means of measurement is satisfactory. Units are usually based on a particular bioassay technique. The unit in one kind of test bears no relationship to the unit in another kind of test.

12

Care of Needles and Syringes and Technique of Venipuncture

Needles and Syringes

The care of needles and syringes is a primary responsibility of the nurse. She may, in some institutions, delegate cleaning and sterilization of these items to a practical nurse or ward maid, but she remains responsible for the condition of this equipment.

Needles and syringes should be rinsed thoroughly immediately after use by the person who has used them. This will prevent the formation of blood clots which might plug the openings. If the blood has already clotted, scrubbing the syringe vigorously or passing a stylet through the needle may remove the clot. It is particularly important, *before sterilization,* to inspect the inside of the needle hub and shaft to make sure no clotted blood is present. Should a needle containing clotted blood be sterilized and subsequently used for venipuncture, the clot may become dislodged and enter the patient's vein.

Although sterile, it is a foreign body, and severe reactions or death may possibly result.

After cleaning the needles the points should be checked. The latter should be sharp and free of burrs.

At times, the plunger of a syringe adheres closely to the barrel. It can often be separated by grasping each part with a piece of latex rubber, either tubing or an old glove, and twisting it. If this procedure does not separate the two parts, boiling sometimes will be successful.

Whenever possible, syringes and needles should be sterilized by autoclaving. If this cannot be done, they must be boiled for at least 20 minutes. This precaution is necessary in order to minimize the risk of spreading hepatitis, since the virus causing this illness is quite resistant and may not be destroyed by a short period of boiling.

Technique of Venipuncture

In some institutions nurses may perform venipuncture, although it is usually done by the physician. Usually the veins of the ventral aspect of the elbow are used. The operator should make sure that the light is suitable and that he or she will be working in a comfortable position. A tourniquet is placed around the arm above the elbow and tightened so as to produce a pressure higher than that in the vein but lower than the diastolic pressure. The radial pulse should be checked after the tourniquet has been applied. If the pulse cannot be felt, the tourniquet should be loosened. In selecting a vein, the deeper ones which can be palpated but not seen are usually more satisfactory than the more superficial ones. The latter tend to have thick coats and to roll away from the needle. After deciding on the site of venipuncture the skin is cleansed with 70% alcohol which is allowed to dry thoroughly to prevent the painful results of introducing alcohol into the tissues with the needle. That area, thereafter, is not touched with anything but the needle. The needle is pushed through the skin and the point advanced until it penetrates the vein. Most beginners make the mistake of pushing the needle too far, so that it goes entirely through the vein. When blood appears in the syringe tip, the angle of insertion is changed by depressing the syringe, and the needle is advanced a few millimeters into the lumen of the vein. The tourniquet is then released, and after some 10 seconds the blood is drawn into the syringe. After sufficient blood has been withdrawn, the needle is quickly taken out, and a sterile gauze sponge is placed over the venipuncture site. The patient immediately flexes his arm so that the gauze sponge exerts pressure on the vein, preventing the blood from oozing out of the opening. The patient is instructed to maintain this position for several minutes.

A 20-gauge needle is used for most venipunctures, unless the patient is a child. Smaller needles are less painful but the blood does not flow through them rapidly enough for most purposes. Venipuncture with needles larger than 20-gauge may be uncomfortable for many patients.

Blood that is allowed to coagulate is ordinarily placed in a small test tube, commonly referred to as a Wassermann tube. Blood that must be kept unclotted is placed in a small, wide-mouth bottle containing either sodium or potassium oxalate or both in the form of a dried film on the bottom. The oxalate prevents clotting by combining with the serum calcium to produce soluble but non-ionized calcium oxalate.

INDEX

INDEX

T